# A Surgeon's Dilemma

A Medical Thriller

Craig Martelle, James Toouli

Craig Martelle, Inc

# A Medical Thriller

**By Craig Martelle**
**And James Toouli, AM, B(Med)Sci, MBBS, PhD FRACS.**

---

**Books in our Medical Thriller series**
A Surgeon's Dilemma –
**https://geni.us/MedicalThriller**
A Surgeon's Peril –
**https://geni.us/MedicalThriller2**

---

**Craig Martelle Social**
**Website & Newsletter:**
**https://craigmartelle.com**
**Facebook:**
**https://www.facebook.com/AuthorCraigMartelle/**
**Amazon:**
**https://www.amazon.com/stores/Craig-Martelle/author/B01AQVF3ZY**

This book is a work of fiction.



The characters, organizations, and events portrayed in this novel are either products of the authors' imagination or are used fictitiously. Sometimes both.



Version 1.0

Cover by Juan Padron

Editing by Mia with LKJ Books (lkjbooks.com)

Published by Craig Martelle, Inc

PO Box 10235, Fairbanks, Alaska

United States of America

# Contents

# Dedication

WE DEDICATE THIS BOOK to our mutual grandchildren – Maya and Lochlan, and their parents, Craig's son and Jim's daughter. We also thank our wives who put up with us still working even though we're both retired.

***A Surgeon's Dilemma* team includes:**

**Beta Readers and Proofreaders - with my deepest gratitude!**

James Caplan
Kelly O'Donnell
John Ashmore
Sheryl Recinos, MD
Lorene Ward
Diane L. Smith

---

# CHAPTER ONE – ROUTINE

**SYDNEY**

"Really?" The surgeon stared at the schedule posted to the operating room wall. It was yet another part of his routine over which he thought he had full control.

He'd prepped for three procedures on the day, this being the first because he wasn't sure how long it would take, but one additional operation had been added. "One hour for a partial liver resection? How did this get on the schedule? Why? Who hates me?"

The operating room nurse had already scrubbed for surgery. She held her gloved hands in the air and gave the only answer that made sense. "It's clearly an error. You should probably ignore it since you approve everything on your schedule." She pointed at the patient on the table. "Say hello to Miss Jean Carew."

The surgeon, Doctor Chip McClure, couldn't read the expression hidden behind the nurse's mask. Crow's feet at the corners of her eyes marked a person with a ready smile and quick laugh. She was pranking him. Her small effort to bring light into everyone's day.

It was Chip's turn to be the focus of a harmless joke with a real purpose. Focus on the patient at hand. Nothing else mattered until the surgery was finished.

"I'm not getting a liver operation," the patient said slowly in her American accent. "It's just my stomach." She couldn't remember the exact terminology.

The anesthetist, also called an anesthesiologist, Doctor 'Possum' Joe Chambers, patted her arm. "You're here for a betterectomy. I saw it on your chart." The two had met earlier. He knew very well what procedure she was there for.

The surgeon had met her in the morning when she was brought in directly from Sydney International Airport. She had developed acute appendicitis during her flight and was taken to Westpark Hospital by ambulance. She would not be a straightforward appendicectomy, called an appendectomy in the United States, as she'd had previous gynecologic surgery in her pelvis and lower abdomen. The surgeon's nemesis—adhesions—would surely be present. Those bands of scar-like tissue formed between internal body surfaces, causing them to stick together. It was the non-routine part of the routine.

Chip wanted no surprises. That was what he appreciated most during each operation. Every human body was essentially the same while being wildly unique, guaranteeing that there was no such thing as routine. Get in there, fix what was wrong, seal it up. Sounded simple on the surface, but it wasn't, and that's what kept the surgical team coming back, day after day. The patients needed them.

Chip finished scrubbing his hands to the elbows, bumped his way into the O.R., dried his hands and deftly put on his sterile gown and then his gloves.

"What's a betterectomy?" the patient asked, her eyes wide.

"It's the procedure to make you better. You can relax," Joe replied.

"We're performing a laparoscopic appendicectomy, what you would know as an appendectomy in the U.S. You have the easiest part in this. Just breathe normally," Chip interjected.

Possum Joe nodded and pointed. "What he said."

She looked back and forth between the two men.

"You're in the best hands," the anesthetic nurse, Abby Rennie, told her. "We'll take good care of you."

Bethany put the finishing touches on the setup of the laparoscopic instruments needed for the surgery, staying close to the tray to protect it from compromise. She was responsible for the right instruments being in the right condition.

"Are you having a good day? If not, I can wait," Jean, the patient, offered.

"We're set up and ready to go. It'd be a shame to have sterilized all this stuff and then not use it. Besides, you shouldn't wait, but the good news is that we are having a great day!" Chip said with his usual enthusiasm when talking with patients. They needed to know he was capable first, and that's where his confidence came from.

The team carried out the routine 'time out' to ensure that all was in order for the operation to proceed. Jean glanced at the IV in her wrist while

Joe hovered a syringe over the Y-connector of the peripheral IV. He verified that the team was ready to go before injecting one hundred and ten milligrams of propofol.

"I want you to imagine that you're on a tropical island, and there is a warm breeze blowing on gently swaying palm trees," Joe told her. "And then count to ten."

She was already mumbling when she started and stopped before reaching four. "Not a record by any stretch." Joe checked her vitals and announced, "She's out. Vitals are good. Standby." Joe added a laryngeal mask airway, an LMA to ensure the airway didn't collapse during surgery. Oxygen would continue to flow. The health of the patient suggested full intubation wasn't necessary. "You can start anytime, Chip."

"Take a look at this." Abby pulled back the gown, just far enough outside the stab site for the laparoscopic entry to show the patient had added permanent marker on her skin below and to the sides of her belly button. *Definitely not down here* was written below the scars. To the side was another statement—*It's that way*—with an arrow pointing at the previous five surgery scars. *No new scars!* was her final note.

The surgeon chuckled. He appreciated the humor. Twice already and he hadn't made the first cut. Today was a good day. "Let's get to work. Can't finish if we don't get started."

Chip scrubbed down the patient's entire abdomen one more time with a betadyne solution. No ancillary infections allowed. A colleague's patient had nearly died the previous week from a wound infection, and Chip's colleague had canceled his surgeries for a week afterward to work out the cause because it was so unusual in modern-day surgery.

Once he finished the final scrub, Bethany positioned drapes to create a sterile field around the operation area.

Chip held the scalpel over the patient's skin for the tiny cut he'd use to insert the trocar for the gas to expand the abdomen and make the surgery possible. He envisioned where the organs were and what needed to be moved and what needed to be removed. He thought through what other incisions would have to be made. The tools of his trade were on a tray, waiting for their turn.

Chip narrated as he always did as an *aide-mémoire* for when he would document the operation in detail on the conclusion of the surgery. Accurate documentation was important as a permanent record of what had been found and done. Chip had also used, with patients' approval, some of his notes to refine and improve techniques and procedures to assist surgeons worldwide in similar cases.

The surgery continued until the inflamed appendix had been removed and then pulled out through the trocar hole. Sometimes they took more work to get out than others. This was the latter. It exited willingly, or so it seemed.

"You were ready to rupture, weren't you, little fellow?" Chip said to the bright-red image on the screen.

Although routine, the previous surgery had created many adhesions in the abdomen and made the operation laborious. This was the nature of any surgery in an area with their presence. He checked over his work one last time. “Looking good. Let’s close her up.” As the introduced gas was expelled from the abdominal cavity through the trocars, he leaned away from the laparoscopy screen and stretched his neck and shoulders. It hadn’t taken that long. He wasn’t too stiff, nothing a hot shower wouldn’t remedy before his next procedure.

A liver resection scheduled for one hour! Bethany had him going, albeit briefly. He should have known better.

“Wait a minute. Blood pressure is dropping. One hundred over fifty. Pulse increasing to one twenty. Ninety over forty, pulse one thirty.”

“She’s bleeding,” Chip declared. “Increase the drip and prepare for a transfusion.” The trocars were still in position and gas was again introduced to better visualize inside the abdomen.He resumed his manipulation of the laparoscopic instruments to look methodically from the most likely area to the least likely. Chip expertly moved the instruments to expose the various organs in the abdomen.

The air in the room changed from cool and light to dark and heavy. Like the surgical team had been transported from a tropical beach to the middle of the Outback.

No one had gone anywhere, and the environmental control within the O.R. hadn’t changed. Nothing had changed, except for one thing. The patient was in trouble, and the surgeon didn’t have an answer.

Not yet anyway.

In these instances, bleeding from the mesenteric vessels was most common, but Chip ruled that out. He could clearly see blood accumulating around the area of the appendix stump. The source was not obvious. It required a systematic look in separated abdominal compartments to isolate the bleed. Chip was mentally weighing the time delay in searching using the trocars as opposed to opening the abdomen for a more comprehensive view and easier ability to repair what was wrong. But that type of operation came with additional risks that Chip wasn't ready to accept. Not yet, anyway.

Using surgical sponges introduced through the larger trocars, Chip isolated and inspected Jean's organs, taking the greatest care as he gracefully moved the instruments through her abdomen almost like robotic marionettes dancing to the tune that played only in his head.

One could not rush, despite the falling blood pressure.

"Eighty over forty and pulse one-forty," Joe called out. "Abby, start a colloid infusion, please."

The volume expander would provide much needed time for Chip to find and stem the bleeding. Time wasn't a luxury. It was a necessity. Joe and Abby were giving that to him.

Open her up so you can see it all, a voice whispered in the back of his mind, but that was the last thing he wanted to do. Blood was there, but the source wasn't obvious. The small intestine? A cut made too deep that penetrated beyond the appendix? A different problem manifesting at an inopportune time? Chip closed his eyes for a moment to clear them from the noise in his head. Methodical and calm. That would lead to finding the bleed.

He zeroed in on a blood bubble that pushed toward his scope.

"There it is," Chip said, evenly. "A vascular adhesion. Let's clip that." With a single application, the bleeding stopped. Chip washed out the abdomen of the shed blood while additional fluids continued to surge through the patient's IV.

"BP is up, ninety over fifty. Pulse is one thirty and dropping," Joe said. He bowed his head, almost like he was praying.

For a second time that morning, Chip declared, "Let's close her up."

"Counting," Bethany declared to ensure that every instrument was present outside the body. She and Chip verified that nothing was missing.

They removed the gas from the abdomen. It settled where it was before the procedure. Chip removed the trocars, and Bethany verified each on a final count. He closed the small incisions. Chip took off his gloves slowly, one at a time, and pulled his mask down. His hands were sweaty. They always were during and after a procedure, and that's why he was in a hurry to take them off.

Bethany and Abby started the cleanup and preparations to move the patient to recovery.

Chip clapped Joe on his back. "Thank you."

Joe kept his attention on the patient's vitals to make sure nothing changed while she was still sedated.

"No two days alike. Can't we have a normal operation once in a while? A patient who responds to treatment without all the drama? I hate drama. I hate it more when it's real. That's what television is for. Keep the drama as fiction, where it belongs. Who do you think they'll cast for me? Brad Pitt? Tell me it's Brad Pitt."

Bethany pulled her glasses down her nose to look over them at Chip.

"Nice work, Doc," Joe said.

"And you, Joe. You, too, Bethany, Abby. Well done to the team. Watch her closely over the next twenty-four hours. I'll check in with her once she's settled upstairs."

"I'll make sure it's passed on," Bethany replied. She executed the post-op procedures while Chip waited for the patient to be moved. Then he and Joe headed out.

Chip, short for Chips, as in Chips Rafferty. The most Australian of men from a time long past but the thought of his routine still brought a smile to many faces—Bethany's included.

"One hour for a liver resection? Who scheduled this?" she said in her best imitation of the surgeon and followed it with a soft laugh. "Routine? Since when have we ever done anything that was routine?" she muttered to herself.

# CHAPTER TWO – VACATION

**MELBOURNE**

Stephanie Trent stood at the rail with her boyfriend, Jeremy Dissick. A middle-aged couple on an extended date, sailing the western Pacific.

They had arrived earlier this morning, having flown to Melbourne from Chicago.

She stroked the military coin in her pocket, a parting gift from her father, a veteran of the U.S. Marine Corps. He had fond memories of his Marine brethren in Asia, and Australia, but not of the war in Vietnam. She wanted to see the countries he'd seen.

The cruise started in Melbourne with stops in Sydney then Cairns before heading to southeast Asia for the next four weeks. It would return to Sydney after visits in Saigon, Ho Chi Min City, then on to Shanghai, Manila in the Philippines, Port Moresby in Papua New Guinea, and ending in Sydney once more, where they would fly back home.

The entirety of their visit to Melbourne had been the taxi ride from the airport to the cruise ship. After checking in and dropping off their bags, they'd made their way on board and found themselves at the rail, where they could see as much of the city as possible before the ship got underway.

"Best view on the ship," Stephanie said.

"You want me to get us a couple pre-departure drinks?"

She nodded, and Jeremy strolled away.

The pain returned. It had been a wisp on the flight. She had chalked it up to a diet of airport food and the stress of sleeping in thirty-minute slices. Now that they were on the ship, it was time to relax.

*Still winding down,* she thought. *Once that airplane breakfast passes, I'll be right as rain. Yep, right as rain.*

Stephanie did her best to maintain a positive attitude. She wasn't sure about Jeremy. He was okay, kind enough, but he had his drawbacks. She expected he'd eat himself into a coma during the cruise because of the 'free' food, while Stephanie only wanted the pain in her gut to go away. Food held no allure until it did.

She leaned over the rail, trying to relieve the pressure. A wave passed, leaving her breathing heavily. She straightened to catch her breath.

"You're not seasick already, are you?" Jeremy asked, holding out a glass filled with a brightly colored liquid and wearing an umbrella. She took it but didn't drink.

"Not seasick. A little digestive problem. That's all. I'm not very thirsty...or hungry, for that matter."

"Don't be like that. We're on vacation. My record suggests that I only take one of these every ten years. This is the fourth big vacation of my life!"

She held up her glass, and he clinked it. They each took a sip and returned to looking at the city.

Her stomach settled for the moment. She was angry with herself for feeling sick. She didn't get many vacations like this, either. Jeremy had paid for it all and here she was, being a wet blanket.

"I think I'll go to our room and lie down for a little bit. I'm sure that will make me feel better."

She handed her drink to Jeremy.

"I'll finish this for you," he told her. "You have a good rest. I'll come get you when we have the abandon ship drill. Everyone has to attend that."

"I know. It was in the info packet." She kissed him on the cheek then made a beeline for the elevator. Down eight levels to one of the many passenger decks. She had to study the plaques on the bulkhead to determine where she could find her stateroom. They had a balcony room, the benefit of reserving their cruise early.

She turned the corner and ran face-first into a man she knew only too well. "Sterling? What are you doing here?"

"I wanted to see you," Sterling Bower said, not bothering with a long story about fate or happenstance. It would be a lie, and he didn't lie to her. He hadn't for the three years they'd been together. That had ended over a year ago.

"You can't follow me. I'm here with Jeremy."

"I know, but that's okay." His face fell, like he had more to say but knew that saying it wouldn't accomplish what he wanted.

"Excuse me. I'm going to lie down for a little bit."

"You're pale. Do you need me to get the ship's doctor? I'll get you whatever you want. Just let me know." His tone was pleading.

She glanced toward the elevators. She didn't want Jeremy to appear. Her head started to ache.

"I'm fine but thank you. Go get yourself a pre-departure drink and don't forget to go to your abandon ship station for the drill."

He nodded, tight-lipped, and walked away without arguing.

He never argued. He was always so damnably agreeable. The vanilla of ice creams. He and Stephanie never would have gone on a cruise, because he preferred to stay at home.

But here he was. What had compelled him to leave their small town? Her vacation with Jeremy. She felt a different pain in her stomach. Fear. The nightmare potential of a cruise with both current and former boyfriends on hand. She'd ask Sterling to get off the boat in Sydney and leave them alone.

She flashed her keycard in front of the pad, and a new wave of pain rushed through her belly. She gasped and fell against the door. She looked up and down the corridor to make sure no one noticed, and that Sterling hadn't followed her. The pain passed shortly. She made her way inside and closed the door behind her. She stumbled over their luggage, which had been placed inside by the ship's crew. Straight into bed, where she curled tightly into a ball.

The next thing she knew, an announcement shook her awake. "Report to your stations. Make sure to bring the life jackets from your cabins. There is a diagram on the inside of your doors that will guide you to your designated evacuation station. If you can't get to your cabin in the next five minutes, report to the nearest evacuation station and give the crew rep your name and cabin number. Everyone must participate in the drill before we can leave port. See you on deck!"

"That person was way too cheery," Stephanie mumbled. She entered the tiny bathroom and splashed water on her face. Bags shone prominently under her eyes. She didn't know how long she'd been out, but it hadn't been long enough. *Do the drill and get back in bed. You'll feel great after a full night's sleep,* she counseled herself.

Stephanie took both life jackets in the wardrobe. When she opened the door, she found Jeremy standing there.

"I lost my keycard and didn't want to knock," he said. "I'm sorry." He recovered his bearing. "Did you get some sleep?"

"Not enough," Stephanie said. "Let's get this over with. I'm going back to bed once we're done."

"But dinner is shortly after. I thought we could go dancing," he suggested. Outgoing and adventurous, the cruise had been his idea. He wanted to do all the things, like skydiving, riding a bike across Iowa, showing Stephanie the world, his world, well outside of a dull home life. He didn't take vacations like normal people, to relax. He used weekends to expend every last bit of energy he built up during the week. "Give it a try."

A new wave of pain coursed through her. She closed her eyes and did her best not to double over. "No dancing for me." She started to wonder if her problems were from stress. She'd heard that life was worth living when it extended beyond one's comfort zone. She had stepped outside hers and found excitement. Briefly. Then she kept striding briskly away until she found herself in unknown territory. She couldn't find the grounding she'd spent her life embracing. "No. I'm going back to bed. Once I feel better, then we'll see."

He rubbed her arm rather than argue further. She wasn't going to be swayed until she had enough sleep and jet lag was a long way behind her.

---

**SYDNEY**

Miriam Kiryakova sat in a back office of the Westpark Hospital's private side, attached to the back of the largest teaching hospital in Australia. "Unified International Healthcare Insurance will pay. We only need final clarifications," she told the gruff woman on the other side of the desk.

"There's a difference the size of the Indian Ocean between 'we'll pay' and 'we'll pay the full amount'," the older woman countered. She was dressed casually in slacks and a loose blouse. Her hair was pulled back into a tight bun. The room smelled of lavender and cigarette smoke. The older woman didn't smoke, but her husband did, and it permeated everything in her existence, including her office that he'd never been in.

The young executive smiled. Her makeup was perfect. Her hair pulled back on one side and hanging low over her shoulder on the other. She wore a sleek black dress that dropped no lower than mid-thigh. Miriam turned heads. It helped her to get her job done. She was an insurance liaison, only as a step on her climb up the corporate ladder.

An American in Australia. Miriam was the first, as Unified International usually put their liaison in Singapore, but costs had been excessive and access to clients limited. The company had floated Kuala Lumpur as an option, along with Taipei, but

Miriam championed Sydney as the base because of direct flights to nearly all major destinations within her sphere of responsibility and the benefit of speaking English. She'd built a portfolio of local representatives in the major cities to act as her deputies. Speaking the language was critical to avoid misunderstandings. She had studied Chinese but was barely above tourist-level understanding of short, memorized phrases.

She was happy for the temporary assignment to such a magnificent place as Sydney. A vivid nightlife in an expansive city. It was the ultimate urban getaway for an up-and-comer. All she had to do was make sure the insurance company paid no more than it had to for covered procedures, which meant not covering anything that was unnecessary. It was a tightrope she walked between the attending physician and Unified International's advisory board. Not every procedure a doctor recommended would be covered.

It's just how things were. Unified International had a robust presence outside the United States. It was in their slogan. *Unified International for Worldwide Coverage. Travel without worry.*

"And?" the older woman asked.

"And what?"

"How much are you going to cover?"

The young executive bowed her head and then checked her phone. No new email. "I'll call the main office. If you'll excuse me." She stepped into the corridor, balancing a sheaf of papers in one hand while holding the phone to her ear with the other.

A young man answered her call. "Unified International, twenty-four/seven hotline. Your name and employee number, please."

"Kiryakova, six one four seven two three."

"Miriam. What can we help you with?"

"Case: Australia five five one one one three six nine. Please confirm coverage amount and specifics."

"Surgery is eighty percent, testing is eighty percent, medications are one hundred percent, rehabilitation is a hundred percent. I'll forward the specifics in an email."

"Generous," Miriam deadpanned and ended the call.

She returned to the office and passed on the information. "That will leave the patient liable for a not-insignificant sum," the old woman warned.

"So, you'll proceed with the operation?" Miriam wondered.

"They did it this morning. Sometimes we have to do the right thing, regardless of confirming if we'll get paid or not. We can always sue your company if you shortchange us."

"I would expect no less. Americans, and other international clients, getting healthcare in Australia is a wondrous thing. We are honored to play a part in that." She smiled. "Happy to be of assistance. Do you know what room the patient is in?"

"I do." The older woman leaned back and crossed her arms.

"Would you share the room number with me?" Miriam pressed.

"I want to say no because of privacy, but she is your client." She waited for a moment before continuing. "Eight Forty-One."

"You are very kind. Thank you." Miriam walked out, steps firm and confident in spite of the three-inch heels.

She navigated the corridors with practiced ease to find herself at the elevators. Up to the eighth floor and down the hall past the nurse's station.

Inside the shared room, she found her client at the bed closest to the door. She was asleep. Miriam waited for two minutes, but there was no doubt the patient was resting. She needed it. Miriam would be back later, before visiting hours ended.

She spent a great deal of time in this hospital, as well as the many others in the Sydney metropolis. Most insurance claims were handled by email and online forms. That's what made Unified International Healthcare so unique and effective. They didn't pay full price and then negotiated the patient's share, sometimes to zero. Happy customers made for the highest rating in the industry. More contracts with healthy clients at lower costs led to higher profitability.

Miriam Kiryakova more than earned her salary. She had earned a stock bonus for accepting this assignment. It was temporary, but it would lead to a promotion, maybe even a regional management position instead of liaison. Helping the sick, healing the injured, and encouraging clients to live a healthy lifestyle.

All in a day's work.

Miriam tiptoed out of the room and walked casually to the elevator. She took it to the Uber pick up point and went to the condo that the insurance company had leased for a year. It also doubled as her office, equipped with filing cabinets, a high-capacity printer, and computer suite that would make any small company envious. When they needed something, they needed it right now. There couldn't be any holdups. No running to the office.

She had an admirable wardrobe in the upper level of the condo, which had a balcony that overlooked the ANZAC bridge. Desirable. Close to public transport. Centrally located, mostly. Downtown among the high-rises might have been a little more central, but the cost would have skyrocketed.

The company wasn't frivolous. She could spend an extra fifteen minutes on a bus or light rail each day rather than pay downtown prices, plus she'd still have to travel. Her current condo was a reasonable compromise.

Miriam went about her job as best she could. A self-starter with boundless initiative, she would earn her promotion. There was no doubt about that. She hummed as she left the hospital for the nearby light rail station. She had a stop she could make before a dinner date with a nice-looking intern. Then she'd return to the hospital to see her client, which would avoid post-dinner extracurriculars, just in case she didn't like him. If she did, they'd arrange a second date.

# CHAPTER THREE – RELATIONS

**SYDNEY**

Chip finished the day with a flourish. The last procedure had been canceled. The patient, a man in his sixties, had missed his early admission. When the nurse tried to contact him, she was told he'd gone on a walkabout, a journey of self-discovery to decide what he needed to do. When he returned, he had canceled on the morning of the procedure.

Chip couldn't force any patient to have a procedure, even if it was lifesaving. The patient had the final say. Sometimes, they just wanted to be left alone to go in peace. Chip couldn't understand that, but he could respect it. Everyone eventually died, but some passed away sooner than necessary.

This man was to have a simple inguinal hernia repair for a long-standing hernia that had recently been showing symptoms and signs of bowel strangulation, where part of the digestive system was trapped within the hernia and being pinched. A very simple but emergent procedure, commonplace in present day. It was a death sentence in past times if not fixed. There was no reason to reject surgery that had a nearly perfect success rate.

Still, people had their foibles. And Chip was able to knock off early. He headed for a light rail to get him to Circular Quay, where a ferry would take him to Vaucluse, an up-market Sydney suburb where he lived a comfortable life. When he wasn't at the hospital, he didn't come into the city. He preferred the more relaxed beach-side life where he lived. The hospital was a rush of energy. He used public transportation to give him time to wind down. It required minimal thought. He could read and listen to a variety of music. The sea air also served to blow away any 'cobwebs.'

The total transit took less than an hour. It would take the same amount of time if he drove, but he would have had to concentrate on driving. He preferred it this way.

His phone rang. He didn't like taking work calls on public transit, but sometimes, they couldn't wait.

"Chip. It's Bethany. Your cancellation? It wasn't temporary like we'd hoped. He's canceled completely. He's going to explore a holistic remedy."

"Although I don't agree, his decision is near-final. I'll call him tomorrow after he's had a chance to contemplate his own death. He might be more amenable to doing the right thing after a good night's sleep."

"Of course. See you tomorrow, Doctor."

"Until tomorrow. I'll bring the coffee."

"Flat white, extra-large, one sugar," she said.

"As you wish." Dead silence followed.

Chip looked at the screen to ensure the call had ended. He tucked his phone back into his pocket and glanced at the other passengers. Nearly all of them were immersed in their phones. A much older woman looked out the window while clutching her purse with both hands.

He renewed gazing at the outdoors. Modern society was in a transition. Life happened out there, but with the advent of social media, too many thought life happened on the small device in their hands.

Chip could see them traveling to exotic places with the only goal of recording themselves to share, to spread influence. He could understand a person's need for approval, but approval from strangers in the form of 'likes' seemed fatuous. It wasn't real, and that was the world into which many of these people descended.

Good people. Day after day, it was the same. Maybe tomorrow, he'd drive and avoid this. If he started reading, it would look like he, too, had succumbed to the evils within the box, when he would only partake of its conveniences. A book, in his pocket. If he finished it, there would be another without the bulk of a second paperback. A full library at his command.

He surrendered and opened his book, a post-apocalyptic novel set in Alaska. He could visit exotic locations through his imagination spurred by an author's words. He looked up one last time. The old woman's grip on her purse had grown so intense, her knuckles were white. Her head jerked from spasms that raged through her body.

Chip put his phone away and worked his way to his fellow passenger. After bumping past, a young man released a profane-laced mini tirade at the good doctor, who only said, "Sorry, excuse me." He didn't bother to say what for.

When he reached the woman, her complexion was pale, gray even. She was struggling to breathe.

"I'm a doctor," he told her. He was a GI surgeon, not a cardiologist, but his immediate suspicion was that she was having a heart attack. "Are you under the care of a cardiologist?"

Her mouth worked, but she couldn't speak. She nodded weakly.

Chip shook a young woman in the seat behind. "Call zero-zero-zero and have them meet us at the next station. A possible heart attack. Please hurry." In an emergency, it's important to single out someone and make them personally responsible for the phone call. Just shouting out for someone to call an ambulance gives the task to no one. Too many didn't want to get involved. Others simply didn't care. Those who did care might think someone else was making the call.

Chip quickly checked her pulse. He expected her blood pressure would be high, too high, but he didn't have a cuff to check.

"Do you have Anginine?" Chip asked, the Australian trade name for nitroglycerine. The woman tried to push her purse at him but couldn't loosen her fingers. He pulled it free and dug inside, looking for a small bottle or a pill case. Her purse was stuffed, just like his wife's. It was a place where a mother carried everything necessary for wiping noses to snacking to fixing a broken plate.

She gasped and slapped at her purse as if trying to take it back from a would-be robber. "I'm looking for your Anginine." He moved into the aisle and leaned over to spread out the contents of her purse on the seat. The small bottle, clearly labeled, tumbled into the pile.

He pulled out one pill. “Put this under your tongue and let it dissolve. It’ll help. An ambulance is on the way.” He locked eyes with the young woman. She nodded and held up her phone, showing the 000 number. He gestured for her to hold it to his ear while he put the older woman’s personal items back into her purse.

“Doctor Chip McClure here. Patient is having difficulty breathing. She’s pale and sweating. Pulse is elevated. Patient is unable to speak and suffering spasms. Patient is an elderly female.”

A voice on the other end of the call asked a question.

“No, I’m not her physician. I’m a passenger on the light rail.” Chip leaned away from the phone and looked at it, then returned to it. “Just have the ambulance meet us at the next stop. We’ll wait for your arrival. I don’t intend to move her out of the rail car.”

The 000 operator replied immediately.

“I’ll get someone to tell the driver to hold at the next stop. They can call you if they have any questions.”

“I’ll help,” the young woman offered, now fully engaged in the rescue operation. She let Chip take her phone while she popped up from her seat and ran forward, through the crowd, many of whom were recording the incident on their phones. “Out of the way!”

“Would you give us some privacy, please?” Chip announced before returning to the emergency operator. “She is carrying Anginine and has a pill under her tongue right now.”

Being in public took on a whole new meaning in the modern era. Chip couldn't do anything about the gawkers. It was the same on the roadways. Passersby would slow down to look at accidents instead of traveling at the posted speed. It was human nature.

Chip dug the woman's wallet from her purse and removed the first ID he could find. "Her name is Margaret Willoughby."

The rail car slowed as it approached the station. The driver made an announcement that the tram would remain until the patient was tended to.

Some people groaned, but no one who was close to Chip and Margaret. They understood. She looked worse than when Chip had first seen her. She was in a great deal of pain and distress, and there was nothing Chip could do besides start CPR if her heart failed. The Anginine was the best immediate treatment.

Except when it wasn't. *Do no harm.* He was obliged to help. Even if he hadn't been a doctor, he would have helped. That's why he'd studied and interned and passed his college exams and worked every single day to be better at what he did. Saving lives was a higher calling.

Like trying to convince the gentleman he would call in the morning about getting the surgery that would save his life with almost no risk. Or helping the older lady suffering right in front of him.

The tram sat at the stop for two minutes that extended to five. Someone shouted for it to get going. The driver made another announcement amid the sound of a siren.

The ambulance had arrived.

The young woman tapped Chip on the shoulder. "I'll bring them." She waved her arms at the straphangers. "Clear out!"

She forced her way to the double-doors and shouted for the paramedics. They hurried to her and onto the tram. They used their stretcher to chase the passengers out of the way. The paramedics collected obs, vital signs while assessing the situation. They began standard resuscitation by inserting an intravenous line to which a Hartman's solution was attached. They inserted nasal tongs to administer oxygen. Chip gave them a series of short observations to bring them up to speed with what he knew. "Elderly woman, likely cardiac history, noted to have diaphoresis and rapid heart rate, gave her one of her Anginine." He stepped back to appreciate their professionalism.

Many of the passengers got off and stood on the platform. The next tram was coming, but it wouldn't be able to reach the stop or pass the current tram. There was going to be a delay. The commuters would have to live with it.

Just like Margaret. She wouldn't be going home anytime soon. The paramedics gently helped the older woman from her seat to the stretcher. They strapped her down, making sure they had her purse.

"Do you want to come?" one of the paramedics asked, "for a warm handoff to the E.R. doctor."

Chip started to shake his head and then stopped. He decided that he better go with her because of social pressure. People were still recording the incident, and he didn't want to look like he was ready to give up on an emergency. "Of course."

He handed the phone back to the young woman. "Thank you."

He accompanied Margaret off the tram and into the waiting ambulance. One of the paramedics stayed with the patient in the back to attend to her needs while Chip sat in the front with the driver.

Chip realized that he'd never taken a ride in an ambulance. He worked exclusively in a hospital. On rare occasions, he had met ambulances as they dropped off patients, but he'd never ridden in one. He saw the way they drove. He thought it best if he didn't try to look out the front window. He looked back at Margaret. "They'll take good care of you from here on in."

He didn't want to give her any false hope and tell her that she would be fine. He didn't know. He couldn't know until tests helped with an exact diagnosis that would lead to her treatment.

The ambulance bumped through traffic while the siren chirped when needed at intersections to clear the way. Fifteen minutes of being on edge while the IV solution dripped regularly into Margaret's arm and the ambulance arrived at the emergency entrance. The paramedics unloaded the old woman and took her inside. Chip hurried after them. The doctor on duty assumed responsibility for her care, and Chip was no longer needed, even though the paramedics had taken charge from the moment they met her on the tram. Their conversation was brief since the doctor needed to order tests and get to the bottom of Margaret's issues. Giving her the Anginine and getting the patient to the hospital quickly had been the two most important things he could do.

Chip had done his good deed.

He stood by himself for a moment. Nurses, patients, and administrative staff went about their duties.

He was free to leave.

He hadn't even gotten the name of the young woman who had been so helpful.

He accessed his phone and requested an Uber. He was done with public transport for the day. Boring had been too exciting. It was time to go home, and he was already late. Nyla, his wife, wouldn't take that well, but he had a surprise for her. Tickets to the Sydney Opera House for their anniversary. Mozart's *The Magic Flute*. The stars had aligned for a perfect evening out.

# CHAPTER FOUR – TRIALS

**MELBOURNE**

The ship seemed steady, but the view out the window confirmed they had left port and were at sea. They'd cruise casually for a day before landing in Sydney. Stephanie wasn't feeling any better. She started to suspect there was something far more involved than an upset stomach, jet lag, and stress.

What in the hell was Sterling doing following her to Australia? What was Jeremy doing on the weather deck? Although there was nothing he could do. Worse, there was nothing she wanted him to do.

"Am I killing myself with trying to keep up with an X-Games fanatic?" she asked the calm sea. She unlocked the glass door and went to the balcony. The neighbors were out and already slamming champagne. She did her best to tune them out and focus on the limitless bounds of the dark water. Sailboats, freighters, and speedboats plied the ocean both near and far, staying clear of the massive cruise ship.

An ocean without whitecaps delivered a mild and welcoming embrace for those who lived on the surface. From recreation to trade, many took advantage of a pleasant day. Springtime down under. Back home for Stephanie, fall was giving way to winter. The cold had arrived, and snow would soon follow.

Another wave of pain in the same spot as before. This time, it radiated outward, all the way to her right shoulder. She didn't think there was anything wrong with her chest. It was in her abdomen. She panted to help herself get through it, but it didn't pass in seconds. The pain lasted for minutes. When it subsided, it left her gasping for air. She slouched in the chair to relieve the tension that still held her in its ugly grip. She went back inside. She didn't want to. They'd only been underway for, she checked the time, thirty minutes.

She sat on the bed and picked up the phone. There was a list of emergency numbers, starting with the room attendant. Fourth down was the doctor. She punched the button.

"Ship's doctor's office, Nurse Arenson. How can I help you?"

"Pain," Stephanie said. "In my gut. Nothing like I've ever felt before." She gave her room number.

"The doctor will be by presently. He's with another passenger not far from you. Are you alone? Can you have someone ready to open the door?"

"I am alone in the room right now. I'm able to open the door. I'll be waiting. And thank you." The pain had gone, and Stephanie felt foolish. In the bathroom, she splashed water on her face once more. She didn't have any makeup left. She couldn't remember when she last put it on. Two days ago, or had it been three?

Her body was rebelling from too much excitement. They should have stopped in Hawaii for a couple days to get their bearings. Beat jet lag into submission through a steady diet of sleep and casual beach time. That would have been better than powering straight through to Melbourne from Chicago and then heading right out on the cruise. She was disoriented. It should be the middle of the night or early morning after a night's sleep, but it wasn't.

Stephanie's head swam with the fatigue that threatened to overwhelm her. That and the pain. She was beyond exhausted. She didn't lie back because she knew she'd fall asleep or descend into a stupor where the doctor's arrival wouldn't register, and she wouldn't let him in.

He probably had a master key, but she didn't want to wake up with a strange man hovering over her. She was in no condition to weather the shock. She poured herself a drink of water from a bottle secured on the small desk.

A gentle tap on the door signaled someone's arrival. She took a deep breath to steel herself for the move. She opened the door to find an elderly gentleman with a stethoscope around his neck and a small black bag in his hand. His nametag only had his first name. "Van" with "Ship's Doctor" below it.

She couldn't help but laugh. "You definitely look the part," she said.

He smiled. "We don't want anyone surprised when I show up. Giving passengers what they expect is part of the cruise experience." She moved toward the bed.

He followed her in and closed the door. "What is ailing you?" he asked in a clear Australian accent. A retired local working his way to see Asia, she assumed.

She held her hand against the upper right side of her abdomen but didn't press down. "Right here. Pain comes and goes. It's too sharp to be indigestion or something that rest can heal."

He had her sit but did not pull up her shirt. He used a small device to take her temperature. "Normal," he declared. He pressed gently across the middle, moving slowly to her right side. She spasmed when he reached a spot near her ribcage, but the reaction quickly settled.

"I don't feel any distension. Nothing appears out of sort to the touch. You are tender but not overly so. I want you to follow up with me after dinner and then tomorrow morning. I believe there's something going on, but I can't tell you what it is. Do you or anyone in your family have a history of gallstones or maybe they've had their gallbladder removed?"

"My mother had her gallbladder removed, but that was only ten years ago. She's thirty years older than me," Stephanie argued.

"A cholecystectomy is a common procedure for relief of gallstone disease. An inflamed gallbladder with gallstones is in keeping with your symptoms. We're scheduled for two days at sea before we arrive in Sydney, so we'll be watching this closely just in case your symptoms worsen." He removed a small packet with two pills from his bag. "Take these. They're paracetamol, it's the same as Tylenol in the States, and try to get as much rest as possible." He pointed to the open bottle of water. "Also, keep drinking water. It's not the magic cure-all, but it does help with a lot of problems."

"Thanks, Doc." She shook his hand before tearing open the package and swallowing the medicine with a generous gulp. Following the doctor's orders. She only wanted the pain to stay away. She already felt better after having seen a professional.

"Get some rest. You have a couple hours before dinner, but I recommend you avoid fatty foods, and maybe avoid alcohol, too." Numerous snack stations were already open. Pizza and hamburgers were available twenty-four/seven, they'd been told. She smiled. Jeremy would sample them all and give her a complete report. He ate like a teenager, but he was always active. He brought workout clothes because he expected to hit the ship's gym at five each morning.

Whenever five in the morning happened. They were seventeen hours ahead of U.S. Central Time. That meant take seven hours from a new day, then carry the one, subtract the color yellow, and cock your head sideways. She looked at the clock. It showed "5." A.M. or P.M.?

The doctor had said dinner. Five in the afternoon. A two-hour nap sounded great. It would give the paracetamol time to work, she hoped.

Stephanie tossed her shirt and slacks on the back of the desk chair and climbed into bed. She set the alarm on her phone and rolled to her side. There was a twinge of pain that subsided quickly.

"Maybe it was stress," she muttered before surrendering to the darkness of exhaustion.

---

"You're late," Nyla said. "Why do I plan to have dinner ready for when you say you're going to get home?"

"Because I'm usually home by then. Heart attack on the light rail. I went to the hospital with her. A slight, old woman, but it wasn't her first, judging by the Anginine pills in her purse. I had to find them in there. That's the stuff of nightmares."

"A heart attack and digging through a woman's purse? You've been punished enough. I forgive you. You know what's coming up, don't you?"

It was a setup question, often answered with a blank look, but Chip was on top of this. "Twenty-five wonderful years with my beautiful bride, kids, and now we're empty nesters. So, if we want to go to the Sydney Opera House to see one of Mozart's greatest, then so be it."

She paused. "You didn't?"

"Don't tell me you bought us tickets, too." Chip had paid a lot for the best available seats.

She raised her eyebrows at him. "No. I didn't think you'd want to go into the city on your day off. I bought you silver cufflinks with diamonds because it's our twenty-fifth on the way to our diamond anniversary. You'll be able to wear them when we dress up for the opera."

"Diamonds? Huh." Chip looked at the floor. He appreciated experiences far more than things, and diamonds were the least of anything he wanted. "It's the whole package. A limo will pick us up at four-thirty. I have reservations at Aria restaurant within a short walk of the opera house. After the show, the limo will bring us home. Is that worth a diamond?"

"Almost." She put Chip's dinner in front of him. She'd been keeping it warm in the oven. Lasagna. He had smelled it when he entered the house. She dusted it with parmesan. Nyla produced garlic bread to go with it and slid a small bowl filled with salad greens across the table. She sat across from him, trying her best not to smile.

That's when Chip knew he'd done right by his wife for their twenty-fifth. It wasn't a fluke. He'd been planning it for a while. He was working long hours, and it left little time for his wife. She volunteered and worked with a number of charities. She stayed busy, but it wasn't her passion. With both children attending university in far-off places, one in the United States and the other in Adelaide, she didn't get to see them as often as she wanted.

The family was scattered to the far corners, and she needed to stay busy for her own sanity.

"What do you think about me taking a paid position working the family support service for the hospital? I used to be a social worker, until Phil came along."

"Where I work?" Chip thought about it for a moment. "I'll be glad of the company on the drive. As we just learned, I can't be trusted taking public transit by myself." He took a fork full of lasagna. The cheese started to slide off so he rolled the utensil to capture it before it strung its way back to the plate.

Nyla smiled while tossing her salad. She didn't eat, while Chip ate like he was starving.

"Sorry," he mumbled. "This is really good." They continued in silence until Chip finished. Nyla took the plates to the kitchen and returned with two dishes of raspberry sorbet.

Chip left it for a moment.

"I'll support you if you want to work, and I'm serious about making the commute better. I ride alone. It gives me time to unwind. I hope you don't mind if I put in my headphones and listen to an audiobook or music while riding. I hope that you would do the same."

"I don't have any headphones," Nyla replied.

Chip pulled out his phone. "First order of business..." He accessed the Amazon app and bought the latest AirPods. They were available for next-day delivery. "They'll be here tomorrow."

He put the phone in his pocket and turned his attention to the sorbet. Small bites to avoid the headache. He found Nyla eating hers.

"You didn't eat dinner, but you'll have the sorbet?" he wondered.

"I'm fully embracing my new role as an empty-nesting adult."

"Me, too, my dear. It's a little lonely, but when you can have sorbet for dinner, it takes the edge off."

# CHAPTER FIVE – RELIEF

STEPHANIE HAD NO IDEA how long her phone alarm had been ringing, but she finally struggled to consciousness and turned off the incessant beeping. It had been two hours. She was deep into a full night's sleep, but she couldn't do that. They were going to be in this region for long enough, so it was important to acclimate as quickly as possible. That meant she had enough sleep for the time being.

She was still tired but felt more like herself. She hurried through a shower, which returned her fully to the land of the living. She put on an evening dress with flats instead of heels. She passed on the makeup because it would take too long. Stephanie found her card with their assigned table number and serving time. She was only five minutes late when she left the cabin.

Her next challenge was in finding the dining room. She headed forward, then turned around and headed aft. The first elevators took her up to the deck she needed. The doors opened to an information map showing 'You are here.' She only needed to loop around the bank of elevators and take the corridor aft, which ended at the restaurant.

The passengers were seated, and servers rushed to and fro with appetizers and drinks.

The hostess showed her to her place at the table.

Jeremy was laughing with the other passengers, looking like he was holding court. When he saw Stephanie, he jumped to his feet and pulled out her chair. "I didn't think you were going to make it." After he pushed her close to the table, he found a nearby server to let him know that Stephanie had arrived. Jeremy returned, all smiles.

"How are you feeling?" he asked with more sincerity than he'd shown since they boarded. He spoke softly. This wasn't part of his usual ebullience.

Stephanie smiled. "I feel just fine, but I have a follow-up with the doc after dinner. Otherwise, I'm back to normal. Sleep is not overrated."

"I couldn't be more pleased. Dinner is a blackened barramundi." He looked at his plate. "Is that a cut of beef?"

"Fish," Stephanie replied. "You'll like it."

"What if I don't?"

"It's included with the price of the cruise, so it's free, as far as things cost from here on out."

He grinned. "I'm a big fan of free food."

She knew that.

"Bare Mundo. Does that mean naked world or something?" Jeremy quipped.

"No." The other passengers had a good laugh. Jeremy was in his element. He introduced the other passengers as if he'd known them for weeks, but they had just met. That was his superpower. An extrovert's extrovert. Life of any party he'd been invited to. Sometimes, Stephanie found it overwhelming, but the rest of the time, she was able to bask in his glow.

His relief at her return suggested he had been concerned about her.

She worried because she considered herself a church mouse and mostly unworthy, even though Sterling had been a good guy, but she felt herself in a rut with him. No rut with Jeremy. Quite the opposite.

She'd never had a wild side. Not in college. Not anytime. Here she was! Australia! And then Vietnam. Her dad would be proud of her. Was she doing it for herself or him or simply caught up in Jeremy's wake?

She introduced herself and delivered her five-second biography. "A teacher in rural Iowa. I'm looking forward to the exotic flavors of Asia."

"A gastronomic world tour!" Jeremy nearly shouted. "Thirty extra minutes a day on the treadmill to pay for it."

The table roared, and Stephanie retreated to silence. A minor stab told her the problems within had not completely gone away. But it was fleeting. She wondered if her mind was trying to convince her that she still had issues when she was consciously fighting them. It forced its way to the front of her mind and occupied all her thoughts. She couldn't remember saying another word all evening.

The barramundi was exceptional. She would never order fish in a restaurant, not if they had beef or chicken. On the ship, however, there was the main course and then everything else. She had committed to trying something new. If she didn't like something, she could skip it and get a burger or pizza. There were no bad choices.

Dessert was a perfect chocolate cheesecake. She inhaled it because they were served in petite portions. She knew the smaller serving sizes were better. Americans tended to eat too much. She knew it. The whole world knew it. She put her fork down and draped her napkin over the plate.

Jeremy had no inhibitions. He asked for a second dessert and was quickly served another portion. "Forty-five minutes!"

The table howled once more. Stephanie focused on relaxing. The tension was building within her body. Fighting it made everything stiffer.

Passengers started to leave. "One level up to the bar and dancing," Jeremy suggested. He winked at Stephanie.

She was getting her second wind despite the fear of returning pain. "Sounds good."

"Come on, everyone! Drinks and dancing. First round is on me." He waved for them to follow.

"Leave it to you to gather a posse."

He beamed with the observation. "What can I say? It's what I do."

---

MIRIAM WATCHED AND LISTENED while the intern talked. By the time dinner ended, she knew everything about him and had completely lost interest. She expected that he didn't even know her last name or anything else about her. She was ready to go before dessert was served.

"Excuse me. I have a client in the hospital and need to check up on her." Miriam pulled her phone from her clutch and checked her emails. She hadn't received anything from the hospital. She looked up to deliver her best apologetic smile. "I need to go."

She stood. The intern was flustered and upset the table when he got up too quickly, spilling the water glasses. Miriam dropped a fifty-dollar bill on the table. He wasn't going to pay for her meal. She didn't want any expectations that she owed him.

"I've got this," he pleaded.

"Dutch. Thank you for the pleasant evening."

"I'll call you tomorrow." He tried to move around for a hug, but she held up her hand, stopping him.

"It's probably better if you don't." She left without looking back. There was no doubt in her mind that there was no relationship potential here. Such was the risk in dating younger men looking for their trophies. Older men were looking for trophies, too, but the risk there was that they were already married. The good ones usually were, until they hit on her and were no longer good ones. It created what she called the relationship dichotomy. Someday, she'd meet someone. Until then, she'd dabble and peruse, like browsing newly delivered tomatoes, looking for the perfect one, firm and beautiful, as tasty on the inside as it looked on the outside.

Men as tomatoes. She vowed to rethink her analogy. Putting it on her mental to-do list meant that she would think of it while working on something else. She was most inspired while distracted with the mundane.

She summoned an Uber, which arrived in less than a minute. The hospital was forty minutes away. She'd expense the ride because it was business-related. She was going to see Jean Carew and talk to her about the next steps. What it would take for Jean to reduce her costs to zero. The insurance company had already negotiated a lower rate, but it was still the insurance rate, which cost more than the actual price.

It was all part of the game. Get enough patients to pay as much as possible while earning a maximum from premiums and paying out the lowest amount possible without leaving the clients hanging out to dry. Unified International didn't want to see anyone bankrupted because of a medical emergency, but sometimes, the worst happened to people with the best intentions. As long as they had Unified International Healthcare coverage, she'd help them get the most from their coverage, but sometimes, they actively opted out of the coverage they needed. The consequences of their decisions could rain down like golf-ball-sized hail. She preferred to deliver good news but was comfortable delivering bad news, too.

Jean's coverage was satisfactory. This would be one of those good conversations that Miriam looked forward to.

The Uber dropped her off at the front door. She strolled in and took the elevator to the eighth floor. Room 841. Two beds. One had her client. The other was empty when it had been filled earlier. People moved in and out all the time.

"Ms. Carew, how do you feel?"

"Miriam. It's late. What are you doing here?"

"Visiting my favorite client. I wanted to make sure you were feeling okay."

"Even with the pain meds, I'm sore. Digging in my guts like they were making a stir-fry..."

"The surgery was successful. The inflamed appendix was removed and should give you no further problems. You'll be right winning at life before you know it."

"I'm already winning," Jean replied. "My mother was gone by my age."

"Can I get you anything? A stuffed koala or maybe a wombat?"

She smiled but didn't laugh. "I'll have to manage without." She closed her eyes and leaned back.

That was Miriam's cue. She had been there a grand total of one minute, but she did her duty, above and beyond. She summoned another Uber on her way to the ground floor. She left the building, climbed in, and headed home.

*Today was a good day,* she thought, even though she didn't discuss the costs with Jean. The patient wasn't in any position to think finances. Miriam would return tomorrow, assuming her covered American clients weren't making waves at other hospitals. She'd check the system once she was online in her apartment.

Her phone buzzed with a new text message. "Insured in car accident, taken to Westpark. Spanish tourist."

She thought for a moment about ignoring it, but she couldn't do that. *Go-getters got promoted.* It was her adage for life.

"Driver, turn around and take me back to the hospital, please. Something has come up."

"You'll have to do that in the app, ma'am."

She updated the destination. They'd only been underway for ten minutes. She'd be paying for the whole trip even though it had just been cut in half. That was okay. Another authorized expense.

Miriam thanked the driver upon her return. She strolled through the doors. The security guard at the front did a doubletake. "Weren't you just here?"

"It's a time loop. I bet I come back at least three more times tonight."

"Really?" He stared at her.

"No. I hope I won't be long." She walked the hallways with practiced ease until she reached the emergency department. The admitting nurse wouldn't let her in to see the patient. They were prepping him for surgery.

"He's undergone severe trauma to his chest, right arm, and right leg. In simple terms, he's a mess."

"Is he going to make it?" Miriam wondered.

The nurse shrugged.

"That's not the greatest vote of confidence."

"We have a lot of blood to clean up. Out here—" She gestured toward a blood trail leading through the doors, where an orderly with a mop and disinfectant looked at it with some distaste. "—and in there. I don't want you to get your hopes up." The nurse paused. "I respect Unified International. You are the only insurance company that sends an agent whenever one of your customers is in here. I applaud you." The nurse clapped softly.

"It's my job, but I thank you. It's all about relationships with the people who pay our salaries and the hospitals that provide the services we pay for. The synergy of our mutual existence."

"Synergy. Of course."

"I'll stay for a little while, see if he gets out of the woods." Miriam didn't plan on staying for long, no more than an hour. She played with her phone, reading articles from the insurance industry.

Forty-five minutes later, the admissions nurse strolled over. She didn't say anything. She only shook her head.

"He didn't make it?"

"He was too far gone. The doctor called it five minutes ago."

"I'm sorry to hear that." Miriam gave the nurse her card. "You can forward the paperwork to me. I'm sure there's a pile of it for this one."

Miriam had been in Sydney for nine months, but this was her first death. She thought Unified International would cover a certain amount to get the remains back to Spain, but she didn't know exactly what she needed to do. The hospital would contact the Spanish embassy, but she'd follow up. Miriam was more comfortable with American clients, but the good part about dealing with the Spanish embassy in Sydney was that they spoke English. She could talk with them directly while contacting her counterpart in Europe. Unified International. They had people everywhere.

Miriam wasn't sure what she felt, but there was a glass of red wine waiting for her. She'd sip it while working. Another client she never met. She'd treat him like she had.

Filling in forms. The insurance industry lived for its paperwork. She was good at it but wanted more. *Keep doing a good job here*, she counseled herself.

Keep doing a good job. *We're the only insurance company who shows up for their clients.* That's what it took to negotiate more favorable rates. The best coverage at the lowest cost. She laughed at her allusion to commercial taglines. She walked back to the entrance, where her Uber was there and waiting. It was getting late. She'd had enough hospital smell for the day. No return trips, no matter what happened.

# CHAPTER SIX – THE SUN RISES

"CHOP, CHOP! IT'S TIME to go," Chip shouted up the stairs. "I made you something for breakfast."

"What?" Nyla asked from the landing at the top. She was in her bathrobe. It looked like she just got up.

"Work. Now is when we leave."

"I said I was thinking about rejoining the workforce, but I haven't even applied. I saw the open position and thought I'd ask you first."

Chip narrowed his eyes. To him, the conversation had been something completely different, but such was the way of married life. "Then your job for today is to apply. I'll leave your breakfast sandwich on the counter, along with the mango that I cut up."

She worked her way down the stairs. "You didn't make a mess in the kitchen, did you?"

Chip feigned getting stabbed in the back. "I have been rent asunder. Et tu, Brute! Then fall, Caesar!"

"Shakespeare. Nice. No one has stabbed you in the back. It'll take a while. Maybe next week. I'll give you advance warning of at least one day. I haven't even been given the job. They might want someone younger."

"Then their folly would be final. Use my name to open the doors and penetrate the sanctuary within. Ho, fine lass! Surrender not to the whims of others. Grip the reins and tally ho."

"Irish coffee this morning?" Nyla asked as she swooped in for a hug. "You better hurry. You're going to miss the ferry."

"Loose the hounds. The fox is running." Chip didn't know why he was in such a good mood. He'd spent too little time with his wife. His job seemed to always take priority. Now, he was in control of his schedule, even though there were more patients than surgery time, it seemed, with the influx of American tourists whose issues popped up out of the blue. The flights to Australia from the States were hard, but were they responsible for bringing these issues out? Never a routine day.

Chip hustled out the door and to the dock, where the ferry was making its final preparations to leave. He hopped aboard mere seconds before they cast off. It was a good start to the day. He looked forward to getting to the hospital. It was a half operating day starting after lunchtime. At first he would see his patients recovering and then catch up on paper work. However, he remembered that there was the outstanding issue of the patient who went walk about. He must get to it first thing and see whether he had come to his senses..

He liked starting his day on the right foot. No matter the reason, he embraced his good mood. Chip would refuse to let any dark clouds affect his outlook. Let the sun shine. *May your scalpel be sharp and your wit even sharper,* he told himself.

---

MIRIAM STRUGGLED TO WAKE. Had she been up too late? Too much wine? Not enough sleep?

All three, she decided. She rolled out of bed to force herself to get up. Her foot caught the covers and stayed behind while the rest of her body cleared the edge of the mattress. She flailed for something to grab, but there was nothing but her pillow. She caught it and pulled it over with her. It wasn't like going overboard with a life preserver. There was nothing to save her.

She hit the tile with her outstretched arm. It crumpled beneath her. Her shoulder hit next, then her head bounced off the floor.

Her foot pulled free, and her legs followed her to the tile. She lay there for a moment to contemplate her fate. "Tile's cold," she managed to say. Miriam rolled over and pulled herself to her feet. She headed for the bathroom to survey the damage to her forehead. One small red mark. Her wrist complained a little, but nothing that couldn't be ignored. "Smooth."

She tossed her silk pajamas and climbed into the shower. She turned on the water while she stood there. The initial cold rained down on her head and shoulders, sending shivers through her very soul, but that was the ritual. It's how she started each day. Most weren't after too much wine and too little sleep, although sleep came at a premium nowadays. She had too many late-night conference calls with the home office. The eighteen-hour time difference was brutal, and it would never do to inconvenience them. She was junior. It was her problem, not theirs, which put many Friday nights off limits and sometimes Saturdays, too. Her weekend was solid on Sunday and Monday, but Mondays were when her clients appeared at the hospital with some malady earned over the weekend.

She accepted it. No one could outdo the Australians when it came to tests of manliness, plus the fauna and insect populations took offense at human incursions. Bites and stings weren't that common, but when they happened, the human came out on the short end with redness, swelling, and other egregious symptoms.

Miriam remembered her first weekend in town. A woman had been bitten by a kangaroo right before she was kicked. Of course she was trying to pet it, even though she'd been advised by the tour guide not to.

The shower warmed and almost reached the temperature of molten rock, just how she liked it. She'd never had a boyfriend who could stand it. That was her true and final test of compatibility. He didn't have to like it, only tolerate it without complaint. It was the last hurdle over which none had climbed.

She laughed. They didn't have a chance.

The water ran over her for a solid five minutes. She'd forgotten to turn on her music. Not that she was in a hurry to finish, but it wasn't as calming to remain. She washed her hair, added conditioner, then scrubbed down with a loofa before rinsing out the conditioner. She turned off the water and stood there, watching the last drops hit the floor.

She sighed and toweled off, folding it and putting it back on the rack once finished.

Two years ago, she would have dropped it on the floor and left it, but that was a different life. She was in an executive apartment. It didn't feel right to have it messy. Being an executive meant living every minute of that lifestyle. It wasn't just a title to put on her business card. It was a way of life. She looked at every conversation as an interview. Give no one a chance to spout their vitriol in her direction.

A high-class individual in a high-class city. She felt better when her place was neat. An ordered mind and an ordered life. Control in all things. Sometimes, her colleagues would Facetime with her when it was later at night. She liked to walk around when she talked. She could do that with a clean place.

Miriam made the bed before she dressed and then went all out with a red, shape-hugging dress, cut low with thin straps. She didn't have time to work out, but she'd get back early and hit the gym that was included for all residents of this complex. Most used it but at all hours. There were rarely more than two people in there at one time. Everyone had their headphones in and went about their business within the confines of their own minds. Just how Miriam liked it.

She checked her computer one last time to make sure she'd submitted the forms properly for the deceased, but they were incomplete. She didn't have all the information yet. The death certificate hadn't been issued, and that needed to be done to finalize the package. The embassy would ride the hospital until that was done.

There was nothing she could do until she had a copy of that document in her possession.

She kept looking at the deceased's age. Twenty-nine. Younger than her.

Miriam logged off and closed her computer. She checked her phone. No missed calls. No texts from the aggrieved intern. She summoned an Uber while on her way to the complex's entrance.

Getting a ride was a luxury but one she afforded herself. Sometimes Miriam rode public transportation, to stay humble, but not when she was dressed up like today. She didn't know why, since there were no appointments.

Dress for the job you want. She would climb the corporate ladder until the CEO's chair was in sight. If not Unified International, then another company. The skills she learned could translate across multiple industries. Project management. Human relations. Corporate identity and branding. Loyalty. Everyone liked Miriam. She didn't make waves, but she didn't allow anyone to steamroll her. She held her own. Debate club in high school had served her well. An MBA from the Kellogg School of Business didn't hurt either. They had a serious program for serious executives. She stayed in touch with most people from her class.

Networking for fun and profit. They kept their eyes open for opportunities for themselves and their peers. Most had their eyes on the top tiers. None of them would accept 'average.'

Without a word, the Uber driver drove away. She had input the destination when she ordered the ride. The private side of Westpark Hospital. That's where the tourists inevitably ended up. She'd meet with various offices to make sure the deceased was properly handled, both in real life and on paper. She'd check in on Jean Carew and discuss her options, then stop by the hospital and see how far down she could negotiate the price of the surgery and hospital stay. She would get something. She was confident of that.

The burr under the saddle. How to be relentlessly annoying but charming at the same time. It was both a learned skill and a gift.

She gave the maximum tip, as usual, to the Uber driver when he dropped her off. Miriam left without ever exchanging a word. Not that he was a lackey or beneath her, but he did his job and was paid for it. She was on her way to do her job. The philosophy of the employed. Let them do their job to the best of their ability. Talking and driving? That wasn't optimal. Pay attention to the road and the other traffic. Sometimes, Miriam was happy being a distraction. When the driver was winging his way across the city? Not the right time.

She took the stairs to the first floor, where one of the offices she wanted to visit was located. It was one of many dedicated to hospital administration. This had a woman she'd met before. Agatha Cornwall. Older and reliable. She didn't let anything fluster her. That's what Miriam needed the most. She didn't want empathy or sympathy. She only wanted answers.

Miriam knocked softly on the door and then opened it slowly when she didn't hear anything. Agatha was on the phone. When she saw Miriam, she waved her in and pointed to the chair on the other side of the desk.

"The answer is still no. We will not take delivery of one gross of anything we don't usually get delivered in a quantity of one gross. Verify with the ordering department and then double-check that, because they're wrong. No one in this hospital needs a gross of tongue depressors that already come one thousand to a box. That's one hundred and forty-four thousand tongue depressors. Thank you for calling. Do not bring a dump truck filled with tongue depressors. Do you even have that many in stock? We're on the same page, then. It's a mistake. Not even twelve thousand. Maybe twelve hundred. I don't know. I'm sure someone has our usage rate for consumables. Yes, please. Call them."

Agatha hung up the phone. She stared at a blank wall.

"I can bring a picture for that wall," Miriam offered helpfully.

"No. I need to stare into the abyss, because sometimes they try even my boundless patience. What are we going to do with a hundred and forty-four thousand tongue depressors? Is someone making birdhouses? I better check the gift shop." Agatha winked at the young executive.

"Could be." Miriam relaxed with the older woman's quips. The best place to find humor was in the most absurd. "I could use some to line my underwear drawer. Give it that hardwood feel."

"You are so bad!" Agatha shook her head while fighting the desire to laugh. "What brings you here this morning? You're not carrying coffee, so it's not a social visit."

"Damn!" Miriam had been too fixated on getting answers to her death questions. She was more tired than she thought. "I need to cancel my afternoon meetings and go home to get some sleep. It was the perfect opportunity to bring you a long black, if I'm not mistaken."

"I'm a simple woman." Agatha steepled her fingers and braced her elbows on her desk. She waited.

"Car accident death last night. A Spaniard, twenty-nine. Covered by my company with one of the cheaper policies because he was so healthy."

"Police report?" Agatha asked.

"I should have thought of that. What if it wasn't his fault?"

Agatha tapped the side of her nose.

"I do need a copy of the death certificate. This is my first insured death."

"The doctor will issue a cause of death certificate that he'll send to the Register of Births, Deaths and Marriages for New South Wales. They handle official documentation regarding births, deaths, and marriages."

"I haven't had any births," Miriam replied. "I hope this is my only death, but I'm going to learn a lot."

Agatha tapped away at her computer. "Cause of death has been forwarded to the state. That was quick. It'll probably take a few days before we get something from them."

"I appreciate the efficiency. I'll contact the police in the meantime. We're not the vehicle insurer, but we do have a vested interest in the accident. What kind of medical coverage was part of the vehicle's insurance? Lots of questions I don't have answers to, but at least I have the right questions."

"And I didn't even have to say anything. I could use a coffee." Agatha raised her eyebrows.

"I'll be right back. You're a peach." Miriam left with her head held high. She'd make a few phone calls and then visit in person. She had much better luck getting answers that way. The police might solve most of her problems. She hadn't submitted the package yet for her client. There could be some changes. Many changes. She'd jumped the gun.

It was an amateur move. "You're better than this," she argued, receiving strange looks from those she passed in the hospital's hallway.

# CHAPTER SEVEN – ROUTINE

STEPHANIE WALKED SLOWLY UP the stairs. One flight and she had to stop and rest.

"Is it bothering you again?" Jeremy asked.

"Tender with throbbing."

"I thought the worst of it was behind us." Jeremy sounded disappointed. Stephanie glanced up at him. He looked disappointed, too.

"I'm sorry. I'll see the doc and get some more paracetamol. If you'll excuse me." Stephanie walked away without waiting for an answer. The last thing her gut wanted was an argument. It wasn't in her head, no matter how many times he beat that drum.

She made her way below decks and followed the signs. She found a nurse at a desk, watching a movie playing on a screen on the wall.

---

CHIP PUNCHED THE NUMBERS showing in the file on his screen. Roo Bantuka. The gentleman who canceled his surgery because his walkabout told him to. It was a basic procedure with a virtually one hundred percent chance of success. A simple inguinal hernia with a strangulated bowel. Free the bowel, insert mesh to cover the hernia orifice , and sew it up.

A rough, weathered voice answered on the second ring.

"This is Doctor Chip McClure from Westpark. I'm following up to see how you're doing."

"Pain is manageable," he replied.

*With alcohol*, Chip thought. "What will it take for me to talk you into coming in to see us?"

"I already told Nurse Ratchet that I decline your generous offer to chop into my groin."

"Nurse Smart, but when you describe it like that, I wouldn't go for it, either. I haven't chopped into a patient besides that first cadaver in med school. That lacked a certain grace, despite my best efforts. I have done over five thousand surgeries since then. I generally only lose people when they don't get a necessary operation. This is a procedure, a simple procedure. We're not reducing the length or girth of your manly hydraulics."

Roo snorted. "I have to admit the thought of another man with a knife close to my nads makes my skin crawl."

"What if I promise you'll never see a knife? You'll join us in the O.R. and we'll tell a few jokes and the next thing you know, you're waking up with a little pain, but we'll give you something to manage that. You don't lift anything more than ten kilos for a few weeks, then you'll never know you had any work done. If you have any pain, that will be manageable, and you won't be at risk of dying from a strangulated bowel."

"Strangulated doesn't sound good."

"I can explain it in more detail, exactly what's going on inside of you, but you don't need that. You only need your problem to go away. The only way that's going to happen is if I repair your hernia or you may die. It's not going to fix itself, no matter how much vodka you drink." Chip didn't see Roo as one who danced around the issues.

"Maybe I'm ready to die," Roo countered.

"Then why did you answer the phone?"

"So I could tell you no."

"Are you telling me no?"

"It hurts, Doc. I saw my pop die of cancer. He withered for years. The man I remember was nothing like the man that he was."

"Left inguinal hernia with a strangulated bowel. It's an easy procedure that I've done a hundred times. Come on in, Roo. We'll do it this afternoon, but we have to let the alcohol get through your system. No food or water or anything to drink until we see you at two this afternoon, okay? You'll feel like a new man in the morning."

"This arvo." Roo clicked off.

Chip could have called Nurse Smart in the outer office, but he preferred to talk to her face-to-face. He opened the door to his office and found her desk empty. He checked his calendar. It wasn't time to prep for the first operation of the morning. He stared at her empty desk.

She strode around the corner carrying a tissue. He looked at her without saying anything.

"I had something in my eye," she explained. A man choosing death over an easy operation was never without its cost. Why had this one hit Bethany so hard?

"Sorry. Not seeing you at your desk was out of the ordinary. I thought you might have been kidnapped, taken far out to sea, where you entered an evil villain's underwater lair as his personal attendant because he's stricken with Munchausen's Syndrome."

Bethany's mouth fell open and she stared. "Did you get dropped on your head when you were a baby? Let me clarify that. How many *times* were you dropped on your head as a baby?"

"None that I know of. Good. You're not in an underwater lair. I need you to add Roo Bantuka back into the schedule as last case for this afternoon".

"Will this be overtime. Just when I thought I wouldn't have money for Christmas," Bethany joked. "That's good to hear that you talked him into it. I thought he was lost."

Chip smiled. That had been a victory. "I better let Nyla know." Chip returned to his office and made the call.

"Checking up on me to see whether I turned in my application or not?"

"Yes and no. Pop-up emergency procedure late this afternoon. I won't be home until late. I thought we might lose one who opted out of a simple surgery, but we talked him back into it. If everything goes to plan, I should be home by eight."

"When does everything go according to plan?"

That was Chip's running joke. Every routine was anything but. "This one will," Chip promised. "I will make it so through force of will alone."

"Sure. I'll get dinner before the operation. You know you shouldn't eat late at night. We're not living in Spain."

"Restaurants don't even open until ten!" Chip and Nyla had gone on vacation there last year. Starting dinner at ten had been too much. It made them feel far older than they were. They were no longer the hip youth. "I'll grab something from the cafeteria. See you tonight, love. Where would I be without you?"

"Unemployed in Greenland?" she ventured, quoting from their quirky favorite movie.

"Too true." He ended the call. "Beth, I'm cleared for tonight. Let's set it up. Inform Joe and Abby. I hope they can stay back. I like our team as it is. The foursome rolls up to the first tee, ready to set a course record."

"If it's not cricket, you're wasting your time with sports analogies. I don't get them."

"Not golf? Not football?"

"No. Who has time for that nonsense?"

"You attack the institutions that have made this country great!" Chip argued. "I'm appalled, with a capital A. The end is nigh! Your subjects have rebelled, majesty." Chip was on a Shakespeare kick and refused to feel bad about it.

"You are a strange man, Chip. How long have I known you? Fifteen years? You're getting weirder by the minute. Are you eating enough fiber?"

Bethany Smart could hold her own in any crowd. She listened more than she talked, but when she did speak, it was best to listen. "Do you think Roo is going to come in?"

Chip didn't hesitate. "It sounded like it to me. I have no reason to think that he won't. He realizes that he might have a lingering and painful death like his father. That scares him. Yes. I'm sure he'll come in."

Bethany nodded. "We're in Two today. I'll get everything ready. See you there." She always walked like she had a purpose. Operating Room Number Two. It was identical to Number One. Familiarity helped the surgical team.

She didn't stroll or meander. Walking was a means to an end, nothing more. Yet, she had a great sense of humor. Roo had called her Nurse Ratchet. Being cool and efficient was a far cry from being cold and cruel.

As a co-worker and confidant, Bethany was second to none. Her and her husband were two of Chip and Nyla's best friends. No wonder they all went to cricket matches but no other sporting events. He hadn't thought about it before now. For fifteen years, he hadn't realized the only sport she liked was cricket. He'd have to ask her why. Dig deeper into that morass of ancient history.

Her husband was also a surgeon, but pediatric. Some of his cases were heartbreaking. Injured children or genetic abnormalities. The small bodies. Chip had his share of pediatric cases, but he knew that he couldn't do it full-time. The Smart family was filled with saints, in Chip's opinion.

He opened the files on his computer relating to the two operations on the day. He reviewed the tests, images from MRI and CT scans. Anything and everything. He searched online for new academic research covering these specific operations but found nothing since the last paper he co-authored on vagal nerve blocking as an option for treating obese patients with Type 2 diabetes. Options. Chip loved having them.

If there was only one choice, that was no option at all. Have surgery or not. That's like holding a gun to patient's head. It was how Roo Bantuka felt, but in his case, he was out of options. Fix it now with mesh or let him die. Chip wasn't good with that. He couldn't give up on the man. Roo had a lot of life remaining, if only...

Chip jerked his attention to the matter at hand. Two surgeries this morning and then one early evening. In between, he'd work on his next paper. There was always something more that could be studied and discussed. Medical intervention was forever evolving. Staying up on the latest was what professionals did. It was due diligence.

It was about choices to give patients the best chance at a complete recovery and a return to a better life from before they had problems.

It was doing something that mattered to the best of his ability.

---

MIRIAM STOPPED BY JEAN'S room to see how she was doing.

"I feel so much better. I have my appetite back. When's lunch? Even hospital food sounds good." Jean adjusted herself to sit up straighter. "I think I'm on a good path now, and the doctor didn't give me any new scars because he went through the old ones. I'm feeling better by the minute. They said I should be out of here this afternoon and enjoying the twenty-four degrees, whatever that means. I don't see any snow."

Miriam smiled warmly while patting her client's arm. "You sound so much better. Last night, you were pretty out of it." She took a step back so she wasn't crowding the bed. "To be honest, I think in Fahrenheit. I don't get the whole Celsius thing, but I do know that thirty-eight C is a hundred degrees and downright toasty. More is hotter, less is not. I like it at thirty, which is mid-eighties. Anything less? That's what hot showers are for."

"You and me both, sister," Jean said. She looked older than she was. She sounded younger. Her voice and her words suggested she wasn't much older than Miriam.

People aged differently. Some had harder lives. Some were gifted with good genes. Others were penalized with slow metabolisms. People were dealt different hands in life. They had to make the most of what was in their control—like physical fitness and diet. Neither of which had anything to do with an appendix. No one was really sure what purpose it served except to cause problems for no good reason whatsoever.

Miriam decided not to broach the finances with Jean. She looked and sounded better, but she was far from healthy. The stress of insurance wasn't something Miriam wanted to drop on her head. Billing and payments could wait.

"Keep your head up, Jean, and enjoy the rest of your vacation. It wasn't the best way to start, but you'll be back on your way later this afternoon, it sounds like. Don't overdo it. Nothing personal, but we don't want to see you back in here."

Jean held out her hand. "Nothing personal, I don't want a return trip to the E.R. Nice meeting you, Miriam."

The two women shook hands, and Miriam walked out, confidence in every step. She stopped in the waiting room and made a call. "Please send two dozen bagel sandwiches, a variety of meats and vegetarian, to the emergency room at Westpark Hospital, please. I have an account with you. Kiryakova, Miriam. Later today? Sounds great and thank you."

Take care of those who served her clients. She'd send something to the surgical team, too. Chip McClure and his people. No one turned down food, and maintaining good relations with the hospital staff was part of her job.

Miriam didn't abuse her expense account. She appreciated it too much to risk losing it. She made enough money to not have to milk a few dollars here or there. She was playing the long game. Serve with integrity, diligence, and loyalty and she would be rewarded. The next level up received stock options as part of their pay packages. That's where the real money was made.

Miriam followed the hallway to the elevator and headed down. She found the floor where Chip's office was located, but there was no one home. She suspected they were in surgery. She wouldn't wait. She had five calls to make to Unified International reps in Manila, Taipei, Kuala Lumpur, Auckland, and Singapore to coordinate minor issues with covered clients. She also had to stop by the Spanish embassy. What would they need from her?

She ordered a long black coffee and found a quiet corner in the cafeteria. She set up a laptop computer before scrolling her address book for the numbers. One by one, she knocked down the tasks on her to-do list. Each call was easy. The country liaisons had engaging accents while being extremely articulate. She thought most of them spoke English better than she did.

Communication was her business. It said healthcare coverage on her card, but the only way to have the right coverage was by getting a risk evaluation ahead of time, then base your coverage off that. Thorough medical exams and tests were included. Insurance without any tests or risk analysis? They would find ways not to pay. They were betting on your health, not your injury or illness. Unified Healthcare positioned themselves to provide premier coverage to every client. It came at a price, but the long-term benefit would far outweigh the monthly premiums.

One accident or illness was all it would take to change the trajectory of someone's life, and not in a good way. Insurance. Miriam was convinced it was worth the price people paid. She saw the benefits of good coverage and the problems when coverage was lacking.

# CHAPTER EIGHT – TRIANGLE

STEPHANIE FELT THE PAIN coming on. It built slowly until it stabbed her right below her ribs. She bent over, just far enough to relieve the worst of it. She wasn't getting better, despite popping paracetamol like it was candy. The sea air should have calmed her nerves. The slightly rolling sea. A blue sky. The dark blue of the deep water. Few whitecaps. The sound of the ship's engines below. And the stack above belching wispy smoke from the diesel power plants.

It should have been bliss. A once-in-a-lifetime trip.

Maybe it was in her head. Did she not deserve a small bit of joy?

"What do you think? Casino?" Jeremy asked.

"I'm trying to take in as much sea air as my body can handle. When we get back to Iowa, there won't be any. This is our one shot."

"There will be more. A Mediterranean cruise. Maybe a cruise around Iceland. We're in it for the long haul, baby! I'll be in the casino. Next deck down. Poker is calling my name." Jeremy kissed her on the cheek before leaving her standing on the deck, leaning on the rail.

She closed her eyes and took deep breaths, but she cut them short to avoid aggravating whatever was bothering her. The ship would pull into Sydney tomorrow evening. The doctor said they could remove her early if needed because the ship had a helicopter landing pad for just such emergencies.

Stephanie couldn't imagine the cost of such a thing, and she couldn't imagine feeling that sick. Getting medevaced off the cruise ship, after less than two days. No. It was inconceivable.

"You don't look well. Do you need to see the doctor again? Where's Jeremy?" Sterling asked.

"He's playing poker. I've already seen the doctor twice. First time, it helped, but now, not so much. What are you doing here?"

"I don't like him," Sterling blurted.

"I figured that part. But you don't spend a fortune to trail after your ex-girlfriend like a lost puppy. You really shouldn't be here." Her abdomen spasmed with a new round of pain. She doubled over. Sterling caught her to keep her from falling. He simply held her, without commentary. Strong hands supporting her in her time of need.

"I should go back to my room." Stephanie clung to Sterling's arm. Her fingernails dug into his skin. He didn't complain. When she let go, he wrapped his arm around her waist to support her. She draped her arm over his shoulder. "I'm not an invalid." She said it more to convince herself, but she was rapidly declining.

The pain. She gasped and stumbled.

"The doctor?" Sterling asked.

"Yes," Stephanie agreed.

He held her close. "Your hair smells different."

"It probably smells like yours. Ship shampoo."

He laughed. "Of course. I wasn't thinking." He helped her into the elevator but didn't push any buttons. "Doctor's office or your room or my room, which is near the doctor's office."

"Doctor's office, please. I'm not an invalid," she repeated. "I can get there."

"Of course."

So damn agreeable. Why did that bother her while also finding it endearing? Jeremy was in the casino for who-knew-how long, probably putting on a comedy show for the other players. Losing or winning? She didn't know. He had money, but no one had so much that they could throw it away in a casino. She didn't think of it as entertainment. She worked too hard for the money she had put away. There was no way she'd toss it on a gaming table just to wave good-bye to it.

"Stop," she said.

"I'm sorry. I don't want to let you go!" Sterling didn't need to say that. Stephanie had already figured out that part.

"No, I meant that I need to take a break. Walking makes it worse."

"Not indigestion, then." Sterling was giving her grief for gaslighting herself into thinking it wasn't as serious as it was turning out. "We need the doc to figure out what's wrong so we can get you on the road to good health. You don't want to get to Vietnam and not be able to see what your dad saw."

He knew her well. He had listened when she talked about her dad, a Marine who served a year-long tour in Vietnam during the war. Saigon. He hadn't told many stories about it. It was like he was trying to forget. Most of his friends were, too. They met and locked themselves away for a weekend of heavy drinking and barbecue. It seemed to help. Stephanie hadn't considered it to be good therapy.

See for herself the land that had taken part of her father's soul. Then again, maybe it wasn't the land. The same war fought in a different country would treat Marines the same, turn them into something unlike what they were before they joined.

"I'll get to Vietnam."

"As long as you don't die on us," Sterling replied.

"Why would you say that?" She was instantly angry.

"You know something's not right, and we're a million miles from nowhere. Your boyfriend—" He used air quotes around the word. "—is off on his own because suddenly, you're not fun. That guy is a clown. Life of the party and all that. Steph, I can't imagine seeing you this sick and being anywhere other than at your side."

"I'm not enjoying that part, either, but he's been kind to me. He paid for this trip. I've done more in the last year than the previous thirty."

"Is that a good thing?" Sterling was a lawyer, a criminal defender. He saw the worst people doing horrible things. When he was in trial mode, he asked questions. Pointed and revealing questions. When he was away from the court, he only wanted to forget about all of it by doing nothing.

"I enjoyed it," she said through a new wave of pain.

"You are a terrible liar." Sterling continued to hold her.

She hugged him tightly, desperate for the pain to go away. Desperate to get her life back under control.

"We could have compromised and not gone skydiving," she admitted.

"Planes weren't meant to land with fewer passengers than they took off with. I'm glad you did it, but you shouldn't have to do it again. That's my not-so-humble opinion."

"There's no doubt about that. I don't think I'll swim with sharks either. That seems to be one of the choices during this cruise."

"It's okay to say no to what you don't want, Steph. Or say what you do want. Like right now. You want to see the doc. We're almost there. Then we'll do whatever he says."

"*We*," Stephanie said. "There's no we, Sterling."

"As long as Jeremy is missing in action, I'll be here. You don't need to go through this alone."

"Isn't this your first cruise?" Stephanie countered.

"It's my first time out of the continental U.S."

"Then you should get out to see the world, Sterling. There's a lot of it out there," she managed to say through the pain that was consuming her.

"No, thanks, I'm good. The world I want to see is a little smaller than what's outside."

"Aren't you being super sweet." The tinge of sarcasm didn't sound like her. It hurt Sterling more than he would have ever admitted.

They continued down the corridor. Sterling was almost carrying her as she trudged along. "The problem with us is that you always chose inside over outside."

"I'm sorry."

"Stop apologizing."

"I love..."

"Don't say it!" She stopped and doubled over, nearly flipping out of Sterling's hands.

He dropped to a knee beside her. "Do you need a garbage can?"

"No." She gripped his hand until her knuckles turned white.

"This can't be good," a familiar voice said from the corridor. The ship's doctor rushed to her side. "Same place?"

She nodded.

"Upper right quadrant. Pain is constant?"

"It comes in waves but isn't going away like it was before," Stephanie explained.

"Let's get you into the clinic." The doctor did a doubletake. This wasn't the same man she'd been with before. "You are?"

"Sterling. I'm with her."

The doctor nodded. They helped her up and with both men working together, they managed to get Stephanie to the clinic.

"This makes you a legend. You'll go on the wall of heroes," the doctor quipped. They laid her on a table, and the doctor examined her abdomen.

"What are you talking about?" Stephanie asked.

"Bringing two men on a cruise. It's legendary. It says, 'I'm in charge!'"

"It says I have unresolved issues," Stephanie admitted. "Do you know what's wrong?"

"I fear it might be gallstones. They don't pass like kidney stones, so once in there, they start blocking things up. We might have to fly you off the ship."

"No," she said without hesitation. "It's not that bad."

"There seems to be two schools of thought regarding how bad it is. Mine and yours." The doctor continued to press on her abdomen. "Is there any history of gallstones in your family? Wait, I already asked that, didn't I?"

"My mother had her gallbladder removed when she was in her fifties."

"That's right. How old are you?"

"Thirty-one." She shifted on the bed every few seconds, unable to get comfortable.

"I think you may have peaked a little younger than your mother. Here's what we can do. We can fly you off the ship to Sydney where, if the GI surgeon concurs, you'll get a cholecystectomy, the removal of your gallbladder. Or we can manage the pain and buy time until you can be taken off when we dock. And the last option is that we don't do anything. I'm for option two. A shot of morphine for the pain, but we watch you closely to make sure there's no infection. An infected gallbladder is a serious problem."

"How can you tell the difference between gallstones and an infected gallbladder?" Sterling asked. Stephanie gripped Sterling's hand like it was a lifeline. He looked nowhere but at her.

The doctor looked back and forth between the two. "An infected gallbladder, cholecystitis, presents with more severe, persistent, and often constant pain, accompanied by fever and chills, while gallstones alone can cause intense but temporary pain, biliary colic, without fever. An infection is a more serious condition requiring immediate medical attention. If we start seeing a fever, we're calling for a medevac."

The doctor unlocked a cabinet and dug through the bottles until he found what he was looking for. He put it on a tray with a syringe and an antiseptic pad. He opened the package and cleaned her shoulder. "You'll feel a little pinch, but after that, you'll feel a whole lot better. I suggest you go to your cabin and lie down. No gambling or anything. Order room service when you get hungry. Avoid the sea bass."

"How will that affect my gallbladder?" Stephanie wondered, already feeling lightheaded from the injection.

"It has nothing to do with that. I saw the delivery to the kitchen. The beef looked much better." The doctor smiled. "Room service. You deserve it after putting up with the gremlin inside."

"What else can we do? Water? Whiskey?" Sterling asked.

"No alcohol, please. Water always. Get an extra four bottles."

"I'll take care of it," Sterling promised.

They helped Stephanie to stand. Her legs had already grown rubbery. Sterling wrapped his arm around her waist and leaned her onto him. "How far are you going?"

"About ten doors down is all," Sterling replied. If he was going to carry her, it was to his room. He had no intention of carrying her back to Jeremy.

Into the room and onto Sterling's bed, which had been made by housekeeping. They'd folded a washcloth into a swan shape and rested it in the pillow. Stephanie crushed it when she flopped down. She crawled to the pillow and hugged it. Sterling sat on the other side of the bed and rubbed her back.

She started crying.

"You were always too good for me. You made me think I was a better person than I really was."

"Stop it. That's the morphine talking."

"Hold me," she pleaded.

He moved in close and wrapped his arm over her. "I have to declare that I have an arch enemy."

"Jeremy?" she mumbled.

"Yes. I'm probably going to have to fight him, aren't I? And I'm going to lose because he's fit. You deserve a champion who will protect you." The ship's shampoo. He swore it smelled different, better, in her hair.

"I don't want anyone protecting me. Just a partner in crime. Give and take."

"Anything you want," he quipped.

"See?" She rolled over to face him. "Oh, you." She leaned in and kissed him. Softly and slowly. When she pulled back, her eyes were closed and her breathing was slow and regular. She was asleep.

*It's the morphine talking,* Sterling thought. She'd be gone as soon as Jeremy found her. "And that buffoon won't take care of you. I'm going to have to fight him, punch him right in his smug face." It was the last thing Sterling wanted, and he knew it was the last thing Steph wanted, too.

She was trapped and couldn't see a way out. The last time she felt like that, she left him.

Sterling got up and wrapped the blanket over her. He sat in the interior cabin's one chair, put his feet on the bed, and watched the love of his life sleep.

# CHAPTER NINE – EXALTATIONS

CHIP LOOKED AT BETHANY, who looked at Possum Joe, who looked at Abby. Chip had his arms crossed as he leaned against the counter. He glanced at the clock for the thousandth time.

"Seven. He's five hours late. You gonna call it?" Joe asked.

"Yes. He's not coming. We'll probably see the paper in the morning and find out he died on his walkabout. I was sure he'd come in."

"I can still catch a movie," Abby said. She cleaned up their equipment, documenting the return of every item to the shelves since it hadn't been used. It would be resterilized by the morning or disposed of if it couldn't. It didn't take long to draw the O.R. down. They hadn't done all the preparations because some depended on the patient.

"What do you think happened?" Joe asked.

"He quit on himself and life. Maybe it fixed itself and he's okay. I would have liked to confirm, though, and repair it so it doesn't happen again. We can only help people if they want our help."

"That's profound." Joe clapped Chip on the shoulder. "Better luck next time. You did more than you needed to with that guy. Don't get bent out of shape. Go home. Bring wine to your bride."

"I second that. A nice Pinot Noir will do it," Bethany interjected.

"On my way, you miscreants. See you on Monday. My anniversary is tomorrow, and we have reservations at Aria and then tickets for *The Magic Flute* at the opera house."

"Going all out. You didn't get her anything, did you?" Joe asked.

"I got tickets to the Sydney Opera House. Things are fleeting, but experiences are forever. Don't forget that for when you get married."

"Not gonna happen, mate. I like my life exactly as it is."

"We'll see." Chip remained skeptical that Joe's bachelor lifestyle was as fulfilling as he maintained. Chip's friends were right. He better go. He'd call Nyla on the way. He summoned an Uber to get him to the ferry as quickly as possible.

The vehicle was waiting outside the second Chip worked his app. Once inside, he sent a text to his wife and sat back to relax. He worried about Roo Bantuka. It was such an easy repair to make. Modern surgery was extremely low risk, but the patient always had the final say. If he didn't want the surgery and he'd die without it, then he would die.

"What a shame," Chip muttered.

STERLING WAS JERKED FROM a light sleep by furious pounding on his stateroom door. His heart jumped into his throat. He hurried to the door to make the ugly noise stop so Jeremy wouldn't wake Stephanie.

"Do you know what time it is?" Sterling asked. He blinked trying to clear his eyes. His wasn't an aggressive question. He honestly wanted to know what time it was.

"Where is she?" Jeremy demanded. His pupils were wide and his face flushed.

"Are you drunk?" Sterling blocked the way into the cabin. It wasn't hard. The interior cabins were small and dark. It would have been constraining if one tried to spend too much time inside.

Jeremy scoffed and bristled at the same time. "Is this the best you can do?" He gestured toward the cabin.

"She's not going with you until you sleep it off and then promise that you'll look after her."

"Promise who?" He shifted his body, moving his left side toward Sterling. That freed up his right hand to deliver a haymaker.

Now that Jeremy stood in front of him, Sterling knew that he wouldn't fight him. *She left me for this guy,* Sterling thought. It was a crushing blow to his ego, his psyche. He bowed his head. If Jeremy was going to punch him, Sterling gave him his golden opportunity.

"What are you doing?" a tired voice said from inside the cabin.

"I'm sorry," Sterling said over his shoulder, but he stayed where he was, blocking Jeremy's way, although it was presumptuous to believe he knew what was best for Stephanie. But sometimes, people needed a knight in shining armor.

"I've come to take you home," Jeremy announced in the loudest voice possible.

"Jeez," Sterling mumbled.

A hand rested softly on his shoulder and pulled, slightly, signaling that it was time to stop protecting her. Stephanie held her head up. Her pupils were pinpoint from the morphine, but her pallor was better. Maybe it was the darkness within the room and the soft lighting in the passageway.

"Thank you for your kindness, Sterling. I don't deserve that."

"You do—" Sterling argued, but she cut him off.

"Can you move already?" Jeremy demanded.

Sterling backed up against the bulkhead and sucked in to be as thin as possible to allow Stephanie to pass. She faced him as she squeezed into the small area. She stopped to cup his face with one hand. It reminded him that he hadn't shaved for two days. She looked into his eyes in a way that choked him up. He couldn't speak.

Stephanie walked slowly through the doorway. She glared at Jeremy. "You and I have a lot to talk about." She stormed down the corridor as much as someone with gallstones and high on morphine could. It meant she walked without staggering but slowly, and without waiting for Jeremy.

"This isn't finished!" Jeremy growled at Sterling.

"Would you think about Stephanie first? If you leave her alone again..." Sterling found it hard to finish his thoughts. He didn't want to hate anyone, but a fire smoldered within him. A flim-flam man stood before him, and the love of his life just walked away.

Again.

"Or you'll what?" Jeremy demanded, while Stephanie walked farther away.

"I'll do nothing. Just like you. We'll both watch her get sicker and sicker, each helpless in our own way. I'll be crushed, and you'll be free to move on."

"What's that supposed to mean?" Jeremy continued, standing there with his fists clenched.

The smell of the hallway intruded on Sterling's thoughts. Antiseptic. Disinfected with a scent of some flower to cover up the more intrusive odor.

"Take it however you want. You should probably catch up with her. She has gallstones, and the doctor gave her a shot of morphine. That's why she crashed here. This is as far as she could make it from the clinic. Go." Sterling shut the door in his face.

His heart pounded. It wasn't the confrontation he wanted. It wasn't what Stephanie needed.

He'd come all this way to fail.

Or did he? She was angry with Jeremy, not him. Was it hope or wishful thinking? And behind all the bravado, how would Steph get the help she needed to heal her pain?

---

FRIDAY HADN'T BEEN COMPLETELY spoiled. The wine went a long way toward soothing a sour mood. Chip and Nyla had pulled up a streaming channel, one of many they paid for, and watched a movie they'd wanted to see. Nothing like Indian takeout, wine, and a movie. They even had popcorn. The indulgence of doing nothing was really something.

Time together. Time without interruption.

Chip had slept like a champ. Today was their anniversary and a weekend, so he woke up later than usual. Nyla was still asleep. He watched her for a moment before getting up to make himself coffee. Instead of watching the news, he opted for reading the latest issue of Journal of Gastrointestinal Surgery, JOGS for short. There were other peer-reviewed academic publications that he read, but he preferred JOGS since they had published some fifteen of his articles. There was always a lesson to share or more to learn.

It was a journey, or so they said. One could never rest on their laurels.

Nyla came down the stairs and hugged Chip while he was reading. "I didn't get you anything." She let that ferment. Chip was fine not getting a present. "Except for this." She put a card in front of the computer screen.

"Professing your undying love?" He opened it up. The only words inside were "Love, Nyla." There was a gift certificate to, arguably, Sydney's best golf course, the Woollahra Golf Club.

"Your tee time is at ten, so you better get going." She stepped back to give Chip space to get up from the table.

"Your anniversary present to me is me taking time away from my lovely bride?"

She raised one eyebrow. "I need to get my hair and nails done, and that will take some time. I have only booked a nine-hole round for you. If we're going to Aria and the Sydney Opera House, I'm not going as anything less than perfect."

"Did I say Aria? I meant the fish and chips food truck near there."

She raised one eyebrow. "You better hurry. Don't miss that tee time. Your reprobate golf buddies will play without you."

"You paid for them, too?"

"I guilted them into paying their own way, but I had to call in some markers to get a Saturday tee time. You have to hurry so I can take my time. I'll see you when you get home. You'll get cleaned up and then coat and tie. I've had your dinner suit cleaned. You'll be dressed well."

"Black tie." Then it dawned on him. "Did you buy a new dress?"

"Nothing personal, dear, but I can't trust you to buy clothes for me. Do you even know what size I wear?"

Chip pursed his lips. "I feel like I'm being set up. Small?"

"That's why you don't buy clothes for me. Get your golf clothes on. Your clubs are already in the trunk. Go!"

"Well now, if I must." Chip kissed Nyla on the cheek and ran upstairs, taking them three at a time.

Golf followed by fine dining and then the opera house. It was going to be a great day!

Chip spotted the dinner suit in the closet, proper for a black-tie event. He'd have no problem putting it on for their gala anniversary celebration. But first? Nine holes with mates.

---

SATURDAY WASN'T A NORMAL workday in Sydney, but elsewhere around the Pacific, it was business as usual. Miriam made and took phone calls until noon, then cut it off. She was going shopping. The weather was congenial, and it called her to get some sun. She dressed casually, something easy to change out of should she need a dressing room, which she planned on. It was the mildest of times. Everything was going well, except it was Saturday and she didn't have a date.

Not yet anyway. It was still early.

She took public transportation, because she was on her time and not on a tight schedule. The city anywhere would do. She'd figure out what to shop for when she saw what they had. It was her prerogative.

Devil may care in things like this. Without rhyme or reason, she would go forth and shop. The rest of her life was intricately planned for the chaos of short-notice emergencies. But she had her checklists and methodologies in dealing with each.

Even the Spanish embassy had been accommodating and efficient. Her client hadn't been the first Spaniard to die in Australia. They knew what to do and were able to bypass her longer channels to shortcut the process. It had been less than two days, and the body should already be winging its way back home at the country's expense since they added the diplomatic credentials to the casket. He was, in essence, a diplomatic pouch. Unified International's cost was trivial in the matter. Ten thousand dollars for the ambulance ride and the emergency room. It was better that he died quickly before costs rose into the stratosphere.

Miriam had been happy to report the case closed quickly and requested payment to the hospital for their services. Time cost money.

She wasn't mercenary about it. Miriam never met the man, but he died when others were trying to save him. His remains were treated with dignity. He was sent home to give his family closure. They would not get a bill from the hospital. It was Unified International's responsibility not to badger the family of the deceased for unpaid bills. This one was covered. The only thing Unified would send through their European liaison was a letter of condolence and a note showing exactly which bills had been paid and if there were any others outstanding. The good news would be that there would be none.

Miriam had seen to that. Lock down those tendrils that crawled throughout the system. Everyone sending a bill. Ten different ones for the same procedure. Slicing up the pie so everyone got their cut. Australia was more efficient in their pricing.

"Stop the madness!" Miriam shouted at herself. "A nice dress. That's what you need. And shoes. A purse, too. It goes without saying." She perked up. "That's what I'm talking about."

# CHAPTER TEN – THE UNRAVELING

STEPHANIE'S HEAD WAS SWIMMING. Too much morphine. Too much testosterone from the men in her life. Too much nausea.

It was all too much. She sought peace, but Jeremy wouldn't let her out of his sight. That was to keep Sterling from saving the day again. She never felt more like a piece of property. The feeling of being a trophy was both uplifting and infuriating. More the latter.

She couldn't be sure of anything, though. Morphine only covered the issues she was having. It wasn't a treatment. As soon as they arrived in Sydney, she would be the first one off. They'd take her on a stretcher.

Sydney's lights were welcoming. The epitome of modern society. A shining city on a beautiful harbor.

With the latest healthcare.

"We better go. The doc will be waiting," Jeremy said. They'd had a complete throwdown. She was angry with him for disappearing when she needed help, and she had told him so. He tried to make it her fault, saying it wasn't as bad as it seemed, but that wasn't true.

But he paid for their trip.

She was trapped. Without Sterling, what would have happened? The same thing. She would have eventually made it to the doc, even if a stranger found her collapsed. He would have pumped her full of morphine and referred her to the professionals in Sydney. The only choice she had was to fly off early or wait until they reached the harbor.

She was caught in a torrential downpour with no escape. Warm and dry was nowhere to be seen. Her last morphine shot was at lunchtime. The doctor told her it would wear off in time for the doctors at Westpark to evaluate her. They needed her lucid for the best diagnosis.

Stephanie remained loopy. She thought she might have received too much over the past two days.

"This is the trip from hell," Steph muttered.

"Don't be like that. We'll get you fixed up and then we'll be on our way to Cairns!"

"Don't be like what, Jeremy? Sick? It's not okay to be sick? You want me to make it go away through the power of my mind, so you can go back to being you."

"You used to like me being me," Jeremy countered.

Stephanie nodded. "Crisis is the window into one's soul. You are the absolute best when everything is going well." She didn't elaborate. He was a smart man. He would figure it out.

"Hey!" Jeremy barked at a shadow lurking near the elevators.

Sterling stepped into the light. “We’re almost there,” he said unnecessarily.

“I’m going with her,” Jeremy stated.

“You should,” Sterling said in his softest voice. “Make sure she is taken care of.”

“That’s what I do.” Jeremy tensed. He moved around Stephanie to stand between her and Sterling. He wrapped his arm around her waist to support her but also to show that she was his. It was obvious.

Sterling nodded. Stephanie had made her choice. He was trying to be supportive without allowing Jeremy to hurt her.

It wasn’t his place to allow anything in her life. He turned around and headed to the rail.

Jeremy guided Stephanie into the elevator. Her last glimpse of Sterling was of his back, complete with hunched shoulders, walking as one did after surrendering.

Just like she’d told him to. Guilt tore at her insides as much as her gallbladder rebelled. Stress to worsen the symptoms. She couldn’t wait to see what the hospital had in mind for her. She found the doctor waiting by the gangway with a stretcher.

“I can walk,” Stephanie offered.

“It’s not a good idea. You’ve carried your burden this far. Let us carry you the rest of the way. I’ll accompany you since you’re still my patient.”

“Can I go?” Jeremy asked.

“The ambulance should be able to squeeze you in.” The ship’s doctor looked past Jeremy to see if Sterling was nearby. “Just you?”

“Not funny, Doc.” Jeremy had had enough. His tone broached no more humor on a subject he found the opposite of funny. The doctor held up his hands. He only wanted to lighten the mood, not get into a fight.

"Just relax, Stephanie. We'll take good care of you." The doctor helped her onto the stretcher, where she lay back and closed her eyes. She didn't want to see anyone or hear more posturing. She wanted it all to go away.

Tears rolled from the corners of her eyes.

---

"MAGNIFICENT!" CHIP WINKED AT his wife. "And the food wasn't bad, either."

Nyla grabbed his arm with both hands and leaned against him. "Five-star dining and you call it 'not bad.' I swear you don't even have tastebuds."

"I do, too. They're just not very cultured. Vegemite on toast is good in my book. There are cultures where you'd get thrown in jail for claiming to like vegemite."

She pushed him. "There is not. Vegemite is good, but nothing like what we just had." They strolled the short distance to the Sydney Opera House and up the grand stairs in front to the entry foyer.

Society's elite gathered here for the night's performance. Chip recognized dignitaries, business executives, and other celebrities. The price of admission for this performance had restricted who could get tickets.

The urgent vibration in his pocket shattered the evening's bliss. He had it set where only calls that he had to answer would ring through. Their children or the hospital.

Both children had called earlier in the day to wish their parents a happy anniversary. Neither had anything going on to put themselves in harm's way. That left one thing.

"Are you on call? Don't answer!" Nyla pleaded, but she knew that he had to.

He stepped to the side and checked the screen. Westpark Emergency.

"Doctor McClure," he answered. His face fell as he listened.

Nyla sighed and rolled her eyes. "I should have known."

Chip ended the call. "They found my patient, Roo Bantuka, passed out. That's why he didn't come in yesterday. He's critical. If I don't go, he dies. Even if I do go, he still might die, but he's my patient." Chip looked as apologetic as he could, but only for a second. "I have to go." He kissed her on the cheek and hurried out. He jogged to the nearest vehicle pickup while requesting an Uber on his phone. By the time he reached the area, the vehicle was already there. He jumped in. "An extra twenty cash if you can cut ten minutes off getting me to the hospital."

"Hang on," the driver said. Even though such arrangements were strictly prohibited, the driver accepted the challenge. He wouldn't violate the speed limit, by so much as to highlight himself, but he'd not be bothered by lane integrity or courtesy.

Chip never noticed the cruise ship coming into the harbor behind him as he ran to catch his ride. Such things were commonplace. Tourists would pile off the ship and invade the harbor area, pouring money into local businesses. Every country enjoyed being on the receiving end of tourist cash. It was like free money, an injection directly into the economy.

But that wasn't on Chip's mind. He was trying not to pre-judge what had happened to Roo, but he expected the strangulated bowel had ruptured. He'd see more when he reached the hospital. They said they were calling in his team. He hoped they all made it.

Chip was happy that he turned down the wine at dinner. He didn't want it to dull his hearing for the opera. Good thing. He could lose his license if he operated after just one glass of wine, even with a meal. He wouldn't be impaired, but those were the rules. The hospital took no risks when it came to their doctors. Zero was the acceptable limit.

The Uber driver did his frantic best but could only beat the initial estimate by three minutes. Chip tossed a twenty in cash through the window as he ran for the E.R.

A doctor in a tuxedo heading for emergency surgery. There was a locker room where he could change into scrubs. He had hangers in his locker but never had they held anything as glorious as his black-tie outfit. He changed as quickly as he could and rushed to the E.R. Outside, Bethany had the information on the screen.

"He's in bad shape," she offered. "He never gave us his approval for surgery, but his daughter did. She signed the form."

Chip didn't reply. He had Roo's verbal authorization, and although they still needed the signature, Chip was confident Roo had committed to having the procedure.

Chip turned one hundred percent of his attention to the test results, including the CT scan. His temperature was thirty-nine-point-one degrees Celsius. Abdomen distended and rigid.

"Ruptured bowel. We have that to fix and then we'll repair the hernia," Chip said. Bethany disappeared to gather the right equipment and instruments.

Chip washed up before entering the operating room. He put on his gloves to conduct a quick exam. He looked at the unconscious patient. "You old fool. We could have handled this two days ago."

He checked the lower abdomen.

Possum Joe and Abby were already there, ready to administer the medication necessary to ensure the patient didn't wake up during surgery.

"So..." Joe started. Chip sighed. "How was the opera?"

"We were on our way to our seats when I got the call."

"I was baking brownies," Abby said. "They're still in the oven, which is now off, so before you ask, no. I did not bring you any brownies. There will be no brownies."

"A man can hope." Joe made a face. He generally didn't cook for himself. Others brought him home-baked goods. They felt sorry for him, for some ungodly reason. He could learn to bake or find someone willing to bake for him. Or he could go to the store and buy enough for everyone. He may have sought sympathy, but his friends gave him none. His problems when it came to a domestic life were self-inflicted.

Chip gauged his team's engagement like an F1 driver evaluates his pit team. Each knew their job. Each prepared as they needed. When the race started, they'd be all business. They were scrubbed, gowned, and gloved.

Bethany removed the instruments from the autoclave and checked that they had cooled. She opened each package and verified that the instruments were dry and sterile as she moved them to the mayo tray, the instrument tray where Chip would find and use each in turn with backups in case an instrument needed to be used twice. Bethany placed a sterile cloth over the tray. She'd remove it when surgery started.

Abby shaved the incision area, and Chip scrubbed the abdomen clean one last time. Joe ensured Roo was intubated, medicated, and more than just unconscious. His obs, that meant his vitals, were stable.

After the standard pause for a final check, Bethany arranged the drapes to create a sterile field around the stab site. They had prepped themselves, the patient, and the O.R. in record time.

"Scalpel," Chip said, holding out his hand, and the operation began. He inserted the laparoscopic trocars, starting with inflating the abdomen to give him more room to work and better visibility. The camera showed the insides of the abdomen on the video screen sitting in front of Chip. He breathed evenly, a technique he prided himself on. Don't get caught up in panic or a sense of urgency. That led to mistakes. Chip didn't make mistakes.

The small bowel was obviously distended, with mostly yellowish fluid scattered throughout. A small bowel perforation. The fluid confirmed what the doctors had diagnosed.

"BP is eighty over fifty. Pulse one hundred," Possum Joe reported. He directed Abby to prepare additional fluids and blood in case Chip ordered it.

Everyone looked at their instruments, equipment, and the patient, so verbal confirmation of each report was important. It kept the team members from making assumptions. "Thanks, Joe. Eighty over fifty."

Using a combination of suction and fluid irrigation, Chip methodically flushed and removed the abdominal contents of the poisons that would kill Roo if left in place.

Chip spotted the obvious perforation on the mid jejunum. The strangulation was exactly where Chip knew it would be. At the site of the left inguinal hernia, he found it had firmly trapped and obstructed the small bowel.

"There you are. Routine, eh, Bethany?"

"Love it when that happens. Are you doing okay, Chip?"

"I'm doing great," Joe added.

Abby snickered. "No one cares about you, Joe, least of all you!" she quipped.

"I care about you, Joe," Chip said. "I'm doing just fine. I'm sure Nyla is fit to be tied, but saving lives is what we do." He sounded like he was trying to convince himself more than the others.

Despite the masks, the smell was nearly overwhelming.

Chip freed the obstructed bowel. He trimmed the site of the perforation to show clean, viable edges, and then expertly closed the opening with suture.

"Vitals?" Chip requested.

"Eighty over forty. Pulse is one-ten," Joe replied.

"Start the transfusion. Blood is B positive. Let's repair that hernia so this doesn't happen again, because we always assume the patient will come out the other side, don't we?"

"We do," Bethany replied firmly, speaking for all of them. A positive attitude and confidence went a long way to relieve the stress of the operating room.

"He's not out of the woods yet, but I think he has a lot better chance of seeing his grandkids now than when he canceled surgery the first time." Chip sighed.

They had a few more steps to complete before the surgery was finished, but the bowel was repaired. It was up to Roo to decide if he wanted to live or not.

---

"NO SIREN?" STEPHANIE ASKED.

"Not on a routine transfer, lassie," the paramedic replied. "Getting into an accident would be detrimental to your health. Ours, too, for what it's worth. Traffic in Sydney is bollocks!" He patted her arm. They'd started an IV, which made it easier to administer other medicine later. If no additional medication was needed, being properly hydrated was always beneficial. It was a standard practice.

The ship's doctor sat in the back with the patient while Jeremy was up front, telling jokes with the driver.

Stephanie's head was clearing, which meant the dull throb of agony was returning, too. "Can I use my phone?"

"This is Australia, not the moon. Of course you can use your phone." The paramedic chuckled.

"That's not what I meant. Have you ever heard of Thunder Down Under?" she asked.

"Are those the Aussie firefighters holding puppies?"

The doctor laughed and looked away.

"Close. It's an Australian dance troop. They do their show in Las Vegas."

"Strippers! My mate had a party with strippers once, but those were different. There was no thunder down under. Sheilas, one and all. It was a great party."

The doctor cleared his throat and delivered his best adult look to the young man.

"Sorry. They were ladies of the female persuasion, if you get my drift."

The doctor shook his head.

"I got it. Thunder is men of the most manly persuasion, if you get me."

"I'll have to trust you on that," the paramedic conceded.

Stephanie accessed her healthcare app and tapped her way through to notify them that she had an issue and was on her way to the hospital. She was afraid of running afoul of her coverage. The app asked for specifics regarding her issue. "Doctor, can you type in what your diagnosis was and what the hospital might need to do?"

"Absolutely!" The doctor took her phone and typed away. For far longer than Stephanie thought was necessary, but he was being precise.

*I have been attending Stephanie over the last couple of days when she first presented with upper abdominal pain. Firstly, I wondered whether she may have had food poisoning and treated her expectantly. However, the symptoms recurred and she was obviously tender in the right upper quadrant. She gave a family history of gallstones and although I could not be totally sure I do believe that she presented with clear symptoms and signs of biliary colic. Hence it is highly likely she has symptomatic cholelithiasis. I look forward to confirming my diagnosis once we reach Westpark and get an ultrasound.*

Stephanie groaned when the ambulance hit a bump and bounced hard. "The morphine is wearing off, Doc."

He gave her the phone. "You can read what I wrote."

She closed her eyes, and her mouth hung slack.

"Nausea?"

"Just a lot, but I don't feel like throwing up." When it passed, she looked at her phone. "That's presumptuous that you think I can read this. Cholo-something or other." She pressed submit before she accidentally erased his work. "Thanks, Doc."

"It's my job. I'm happy to do it." He checked her vitals. Still no fever. That gave him confidence that her gallbladder wasn't infected.

The ambulance pulled into the emergency entrance, and they unloaded. Jeremy was last out after shaking hands with the driver and sharing one final laugh.

The doctor looked at her apologetically.

"I know," she admitted.

They wheeled her into the hospital, where they continued straight to a room and moved her to one of the hospital beds. She wasn't there more than five minutes when they took her, complete with the bed, to get an ultrasound, which was the best diagnostic tool for finding gallstones.

Jeremy stayed in the room while they took Stephanie away for her tests.

"America, huh? What brings you to our humble little hospital?" an orderly asked while wheeling the bed down the corridor.

"It was on the list of tours from the ship. I don't like crowds and since no one else signed up for it, here I am."

"That's a good one! Ha!" He was easily amused, but the job was hard enough that he didn't have to be miserable when there was no call for it. Stephanie was in a waning stage of pain. Being at the hospital was a relief. A full diagnostic suite for them to pinpoint her exact problem and then deal with it. Whatever that took.

She didn't want to admit it to herself, but she hoped it would be serious enough that she'd have to leave the cruise and heal enough to fly back to the States. It had been her dream to see the country her father had served in, but the trip had become a nightmare.

So much stress. She was more of a homebody than she wanted to admit. There was good excitement and bad. This trip had lurched far beyond bad and was getting worse every minute she had to spend with Jeremy. She'd get her tests and then be taken back to where he waited. Her pulse quickened, and she struggled for breath.

"Are you okay, miss? I'll get the doctor." He stepped away from the bed for a moment and returned with a young E.R. doctor.

"It looks like you're in some distress," he said before grabbing the chart off the foot of the bed and studying it. "Possible gallstones. Those will make your breath catch. Look at me." He checked her pupils. "We need a couple tests to see what's going on."

"It's not that," Stephanie said, staring at the doctor, who looked too intense. "Home life is stressing me out. Cure one problem and another pops up. Am I right?"

"You know the first rule of consulting? When you take care of the number one problem, number two becomes number one."

"Are you a consultant?" Stephanie wondered.

"I'm a resident doctor, but my father is a specialist. He put me through med school. I owe him, and now I've shared some of his hard-earned knowledge with you. That knocks a thousand dollars off my debt to him."

Stephanie managed a weak smile. "I'll remember that."

The doctor motioned for the orderly to continue. Stephanie had tests that needed to be run.

# CHAPTER ELEVEN – MACHINATIONS

STERLING STOOD AT THE ship's rail on the upper deck. A warm, salty breeze flowed past. It might have been cool, but he didn't feel it. He stared at the city's lights. He'd already purchased a plane ticket home. He'd leave the ship in the morning. There was nothing left for him here.

He'd invested hugely in wishful thinking. He should have just gambled the money away. He'd have just as much to show for it. Impulsiveness was not rewarded. He'd failed.

And his soul was crushed.

"Phone call for a Mister Sterling Bower. Please access the nearest courtesy phone." The announcement repeated. He knew there was no one else on board with his name. It was uncommon enough that growing up, the other kids always made fun of him. He got used to it, and now, he'd seen his former classmates in court, on the wrong side of the trial. He didn't feel sorry for them. They were mean as kids and it finally did them ugly as adults.

Still, he had shown them far more mercy than they showed him. Sometimes as the public defender. Other times as the prosecutor when he argued for a lighter sentence.

They might forget what he did for them, but he would never forget what they did to him.

There was a courtesy phone by the elevators, so that's where he went. He picked it up, and an operator answered almost immediately.

"I'm Sterling Bower."

"One second please. We have a call from the city. I'll transfer it to you." The phone clicked and buzzed until a second click. The operator continued. "Doctor, Mister Bower is on the line."

"Hey, kid, what the hell do you think you're doing? She needs you now more than ever, and she's stuck with that clown. Get your ass to Westpark Hospital!"

"I'm sorry. Where is she?"

"Westpark Hospital. The private side. Hurry up. She might have surgery tonight. It would be best if she woke up to a friendly face."

"Jeremy won't like that very much," Sterling countered. "Us fighting over her won't be what she needs. It's really her decision, and she's already made it."

"Has she? Or is she in a situation over which she has no control?"

"Man, Doc. You're setting me up to fail. Again. I bought my plane tickets out of Sydney tomorrow. I'm off the ship, and I'll be on my way back to America, where I belong."

"What does tomorrow have to do with today? Get down here. I'll be waiting." The line went dead.

"Yes, Dad," Sterling told the phone before he placed the receiver on the hook. He didn't know what to do, so he stood there, staring at the phone and replaying the conversation with the doctor. The kind doctor who had made light of two men vying for Stephanie's affections. The doctor had chosen a winner in the contest, and it wasn't Jeremy.

That might have given Sterling solace, but Stephanie had made her choice, again and again, seemingly angry with herself for it. Yet, she walked away.

"I guess I'm going to the hospital," Sterling said to bolster his confidence and his courage. Public affirmations galvanize individuals to action. "It'll be what it is."

If Jeremy beat him up, at least he'd be in the right place to get treated.

---

A MESSAGE ALERTED MIRIAM to an American client being transported from a cruise ship to Westpark for a potential emergency cholecystectomy—removal of a gallbladder—which should have been a fairly routine surgery.

She looked at herself in the mirror. She had her new dress on, complete with two-inch heels. She hadn't found a purse that matched, but she went with a black clutch, which went well with all things.

"Maybe there's a tasty E.R. doctor who has nothing better to do than take me to dinner," she posited and then laughed. "Probably not. Look at you. Pathetic. Going to the hospital to look for a date. I mean, see a client. Yes, that's exactly it."

She didn't need to go see one Stephanie Trent, but she was disappointed in her Saturday evening. There was no sense sitting at home and moping about it.

Miriam summoned an Uber on her way from her condo. She waited on the street for five minutes, watching the app as the car crawled along the roads to her place. She remained amazed by the technology that she could track the vehicle throughout the process. It was a safety measure. She also carried a hairbrush with a steel spike in the handle. She'd never had to stab anyone, but she would if there was no other way out of a situation.

She had a silent ride as her default option, and the drivers almost always respected that. She climbed in without a word, and they were on their way to the hospital.

She had five clients at hospitals around Sydney, which was a minor number considering how many international travelers came to Australia and found their way to Sydney. But the ones that needed surgery drew her attention because those could result in high-dollar payouts. Stephanie's insurance wasn't great. Emergency surgery could cost the company tens of thousands, but it would also cost her about the same.

A health emergency to financial ruination. She didn't even know the woman, but Miriam knew that she would do what she could to bring down the costs for both parties.

And that's why she was going to the hospital. On the way, she ordered bagel sandwiches for those working in the emergency room. It was worth the cost, multiple times over.

Miriam reviewed Stephanie's file again to see if she missed anything. Single. Thirty-one. They were the same age. That made Miriam instantly like her. Same age, yet one of them was in the hospital on the wrong end of a bad roll of the dice. She decided she wanted to help her. A fellow American. A low-risk procedure, but still important with lots of moving parts.

Miriam chewed her lip in contemplation. Her new dress was already losing its luster. It would smell like the hospital instead of a high-end designer's shop. What were the important things in life? Retail therapy was fine, but she didn't need anything, didn't need to spend the money she was making on things that were relatively frivolous.

She had an image to maintain! She saw different people every day. Westpark Hospital multiple times over three days? That was out of the ordinary.

The Uber pulled up out front, and Miriam got out without ever saying a word to the driver. She left a few dollars' tip as she usually did, even though Australia wasn't a tip culture like in the United States.

She walked briskly through the doors and to the admissions counter. "If my client is available, I'd like to speak with her. Stephanie Trent." Miriam handed her business card over.

"This is irregular," the nurse told her. "We don't usually allow anyone back there but a family member or authorized representative, but..." She hesitated. "She's an American, and she'll need you to sort out her options."

"Ones that cost more versus ones that cost less, you mean? I'm not certified to dissuade doctors from doing what's best for our clients. I do want her to understand what the limits are, depending on what procedures are viable options for her illness."

"That's why I'm letting you go back there. Please follow me." The nurse swiped her badge at the door and went through. Miriam was right behind her. She took two turns and then entered a patient room where the bed was missing and a man waited in a chair. He stood when they appeared.

"This is Stephanie's insurance agent. Enjoy." The nurse walked out after that less-than-gracious introduction.

"I'm Miriam Kiryakova, from Unified International Healthcare. I wanted to talk with Stephanie. Is she coming back?"

He nodded. "I'm Jeremy, Jeremy Dissick. They took her for tests. An ultrasound, a CT scan, and I don't know what else." He offered his hand and a warm smile.

"Who are you to her?" Miriam asked before sharing any confidential client information.

"I'm her friend."

"Do you have a medical power of attorney?"

He shook his head.

"Then I'll wait until she gets back so I can talk with her directly." Miriam leaned against the counter and crossed her arms. Being alone in a room with a strange man hadn't topped her list of priorities for the evening.

"Do you skydive?" he asked.

"No desire to jump out of an airplane. Were you on the cruise with Stephanie? I was told they brought her here from the ship," Miriam pressed.

"Yes. We came together."

"Her boyfriend," Miriam clarified.

"Maybe. There seems to be some debate on that at the moment. You see, her ex followed us on the cruise and has been making moves on her and now she's, well, confused."

Miriam's eyes went wide of their own accord before she was able to school her features. It wasn't her place to judge. No wonder her client was having problems.

The curtain was brushed aside. "Hey, Doc." Jeremy waved.

The ship's doctor studied the newcomer. "Are you from the hospital?"

"Unified International Healthcare. I'm Stephanie's insurance representative. I thought I'd stop by to make sure there weren't any problems and that she received the care she needed." Miriam held out her business card. "Miriam Kiryakova."

"An insurance agent. This night gets better and better. A necessary evil, I guess."

"Do I look evil?" Miriam asked.

"Poor choice of words on my part," the doctor conceded. "I came with Stephanie from the ship. I'm the ship's doctor, Van Liet."

"Doctor Van Liet," Miriam repeated to help her remember the name. The ship's doctor taking responsibility. Maybe the cruise line could cover some of the costs. She made a mental note. "Thank you for making sure she came in. We'll see what the tests find, and Stephanie can decide how to move forward from there. The decision is completely hers."

The doctor looked skeptical. "Based on what you pay for?"

"You're painting me in a far more mercenary light than I deserve. You can stay while I consult with my client since you are her doctor. I don't want any misunderstanding. It's Saturday night. I'm in the hospital because I believe in those we insure."

"I'm sorry. I've had bad experiences with insurance companies and our American passengers. They don't always pay, and the patient is the one who suffers. Stress—" He looked pointedly at Jeremy. "—is hard on the body and makes recovery that much more difficult."

"I understand," Miriam replied. She did. The dynamic with the man was interesting, to say the least. She expected that he would hit on her at some point during the evening. They almost always did. He was fit but had a look that seemed to constantly calculate odds. He thought before he spoke, but when he spoke, it was measured. She seemed to have caught both of them when they weren't on their best behavior.

Miriam felt like she was at the top of her game. She wanted to talk with Stephanie.

"Where'd you go, Doc? The ship food get to you?" Jeremy asked, his face completely transformed from earlier. His new image was happy-go-lucky with a little devil-may-care attitude thrown in.

"I had to make a phone call," the doctor said without elaborating.

"Calling down the thunder, no doubt! Thank you for everything you've done for Stephanie. She was feeling a lot better the last day and a half. Your treatment was working wonders."

"Treatment? Morphine isn't a treatment. It helps the patient deal with the pain. That's it. It does nothing to resolve the underlying issues. But we watched closely for any signs of infection, and she's not showing any," the doctor explained.

Miriam listened. She was a veritable novice when it came to medical procedures, but even she knew that morphine wasn't a treatment. Pain relief could be two-sided. The patient thinks they're better and does things they shouldn't be doing, or the patient likes the feeling of being pain-free and heads down the wrong road to addiction. Getting the patient healed and off morphine was the hospital's focus.

"Doctor, a word, please," a fresh-faced young man with a stethoscope around his neck said. He glanced at the mob of people in the room before letting the curtain fall aside and stepping into the corridor. Miriam was in a good position to hear them if they didn't move too far from the room.

"If you'll excuse me," Doctor Van Liet said and stepped into the hallway.

Miriam listened intently to the conversation.

"The surgeon is in the middle of emergency surgery right now. It'll be a while before he's available—that is, if he becomes available, depending on how draining his current operation is."

"You have only one surgeon?"

"We have the best GI surgeon. He's the right doctor for this job, as long as we determine that she can wait."

"What did the tests show?" the ship's doctor pressed. Concern tinged the tone of his voice.

"Haven't gotten them back yet. I'll let you know."

Jeremy cleared his throat to get Miriam's attention. She lifted her head.

"Just making sure you weren't getting ready to pass out. The smells in a hospital can be overwhelming—antiseptics, antibiotics, and bodily fluids." He shrugged.

"Can you smell antibiotics?" Miriam wondered.

"You can smell when they don't work."

Infections. He probably wasn't wrong. "True."

"You're not from here, judging by your accent," Jeremy said.

"States. Just like most of my clients, those who insure with Unified International." She handed him her business card.

"Is this your personal number?" he asked while reading the card.

"Office," she said, even though her office was wherever she happened to be and the number was to the cell phone in her pocket.

He punched the number into a phone she hadn't seen him holding. The phone in her purse buzzed. Jeremy looked at her with an even expression. "I'm sure that's a coincidence," he said, giving her an out. He pressed 'end,' and the phone stopped vibrating. "I just wanted to have your number in case Stephanie has any questions."

"Of course," Miriam replied. Her instant connection with her client was waning if this was her boyfriend.

Neither doctor returned, and she could no longer hear them. Miriam pulled the curtain aside and found the corridor outside Stephanie's room to be empty.

"Did you hear where they were going?" She pointed at the corridor.

He shook his head. Miriam crossed her arms and leaned against the counter. Jeremy mirrored her pose, a standard technique to disarm a counterpart. Many negotiators used it so one side would feel what they were projecting. It helped bridge gaps in conversations, opening them up to better conversations.

"Your company sent you all the way down here to hang out in the emergency room on a Saturday night?"

"I manage this entire region, but sometimes, there are special cases that I want to administer personally. Also, Westpark is an outstanding hospital with the best medical professionals. I learn whenever I come here. That's part of my job, too. Insurance is far more than getting people to pay their premiums, which I don't have any part of. I manage the other part. What does the client's policy cover?"

"What does Stephanie's policy cover? I can fill in some shortfalls for her, depending." He tried to look humble. He was anything but.

# CHAPTER TWELVE – RELATIONS

ABBY CAME AROUND FROM the anesthetic area and wiped Chip's brow. He was sweating under the surgery's bright lights. Two hours into the operation and the challenges with the bowel had finally been resolved.

Roo stood on the brink, dangerously close to death. The rupture had sent a great deal of poison into his body, and it was doing a number on him. His fever was coming down, thanks to medication, but his vitals were all over the place, waxing and waning with each fresh assault from within.

Chip replayed his conversations with Roo over and over in his mind. What else could he have said to forestall Roo's walkabout and get him on the table earlier, before the rupture? It would have been so easy to fix.

Now Roo was fighting for his life. Maybe get his daughter involved at the outset. But Roo was an adult who was legally responsible for his own decisions. These were the consequences.

At this stage, Chip diverted his attention to the hernial orifice. That was the cause of the problem in the first place. He closed it using mono filament nylon sutures. Not the ideal of repairs for a hernia but in the presence of a potentially 'dirty' abdominal cavity, a mesh might become infected. Best to temporize and deal with any recurrent hernia once Roo recovered.

"That's all I can do. I'm closing him up." Chip leaned back, almost too tired to stand. He waited until the last skin suture was in before pulling his mask down. He didn't immediately remove his gown or gloves. "Good work, people. It's all up to Mister Bantuka now. How badly does he want to live?"

"I think his daughter is in the waiting room," Bethany said as she busied herself with cleanup. Abby joined her while Joe secured his equipment.

"Pressors, intubated, and move to the ICU. Watch for a blood infection. Keep him sedated for the next twenty-four hours, at least." He took a deep breath trying to steel himself. "I'll talk to her."

Chip removed his gloves and dropped them in the hazardous waste disposal. He had wisps of blood on his gown, too. He removed it and tossed it in the laundry bin. He headed to the waiting room but stopped before he got there to take a drink of water from the fountain.

He straightened and walked through the doors. There were a few people out there, but only one looked to be related to Roo Bantuka. "Miss Bantuka?" Chip said loudly enough to get everyone's attention. The woman he suspected was up in an instant and hurried toward him.

It was always a challenge being truthful while allaying some of their fears. Facts usually worked best. Give hope but not false hope.

"Your father is out of surgery. We've repaired his strangulated bowel and the hernia that caused it, but there was a lot of damage because of the flood of toxins through the rupture."

"Is he going to live?" she asked, already crying.

"It's up to him at this point. He's pumped full of antibiotics. His obs are unstable. We should know for sure within the next few days. All he has to do is make it through tonight which will give us hope for a better tomorrow and that the antibiotics are doing what they need to do. I'm optimistic that he was brought in in time. Do we have you to thank for that?" Chip needed his vital signs.

"I found him, yes. Stubborn old fool." Chip held her while she sobbed.

"Go home and get some rest, even if you don't sleep. We'll call if there is any change. And we'll call in the morning, regardless."

"Thank you." She wiped her face on her sleeve.

Chip retreated into the surgical suite and to the locker room. His dinner suit hung on a hanger. He didn't want to put it on. The thrill of being dressed up had come and gone. He'd wear scrubs home. It was frowned upon, but sometimes, it couldn't be avoided. He'd leave his dinner suit and bring a garment bag for it when he returned to the hospital, probably tomorrow.

The emergency room doctor appeared. "Hey, Chip. There's another emergency requiring your expertise. A gallbladder that's acting up. We have the scans and blood results. American off the cruise ship."

"I don't think I'll be able to do anything tonight, unless it's life or death." The round of golf had taken more out of Chip than he wanted to admit. He was getting older, and that meant his energy waned late in the day. There would be no more all-nighters in his life. That era was long past. He wouldn't drink the energy drinks that young doctors and the new generation of nurses embraced. They weren't good for you and would create problems farther down the road, but that was today. Do what they had to survive the here and now. Thrive with unnatural vigor. Accept the crash and then do it all again.

"Here's the information and pictures." The doctor held a folder in front of him.

"What's your prognosis? Can she wait?"

"Yes. She'll still be here in the morning. You can take care of her after you've had some sleep. Are you going to stay here tonight?"

They had rooms for doctors to use if needed.

"It's my twenty-fifth anniversary today, well, whatever's left of today."

The young doctor noted the dinner suit for the first time. "Oh, mate. Sorry about that."

"I'm going home. I'll be back in the morning, soon as I can."

"Putting her on ice. We'll make sure she's okay. Kramer is on call, too, if need be."

"GI isn't his specialty, though."

"If it needs to be done and you can't do it, what choice do we have besides transferring her to another hospital? And you know how the administrators love that. We're up for hospital of the century or something. They aren't thinking straight."

Chip chuckled. "No one thinks straight at this hour." He took one last look at the folder. "Tell Stephanie I'll see her in the morning and we'll discuss options. Give her morphine to ensure she rests and keep her prepped. No food or water."

"Will do, Chip. For what it's worth, happy anniversary. She must be some woman to put up with you for abandoning her at some black-tie gala."

"She is. Better than I deserve. Good luck, John."

"You, too." The E.R. doc left Chip to his own. A quick shower and then a taxi home. He didn't have the energy for anything else.

---

THE ORDERLY WHEELED STEPHANIE into the room where she'd left Jeremy and the ship's doctor. She found a striking woman in there as well. Stephanie's first judgment was obvious in how she glared at Jeremy.

"Stephanie," the woman said to get her attention. "I'm Miriam Kiryakova with Unified International Healthcare. I wanted to see how you're doing."

"You're an insurance agent?" Stephanie was lucid but in pain, though not as much as she was in earlier.

"I'm the liaison. We can talk about your coverage and what you might be responsible for regarding costs so you can make the best decision regarding treatment options."

"They can't just take care of me and you pay for it?"

Miriam smiled. "If only it worked that way. Your coverage is limited in this regard. I'll do what I can to keep costs down, regardless of the option you pick."

"What are my options?" Stephanie asked.

"I don't know. I was hoping you could tell me," Miriam countered.

"No one knows anything. Isn't this delightful?" Jeremy interjected.

Stephanie barely glanced at him. Her attention was on Miriam. "Can you find out?"

"I'll do that," Jeremy offered. He smiled at Miriam on his way out. He turned around and walked back in; the young doctor was right behind him with Doctor Van Liet. Stephanie's room was filled with people.

"Do we need privacy?" he asked.

"No need," Stephanie said. "Everyone has a part to play in this circus."

The ship's doctor held the curtain open for one more person.

Sterling Bower stepped in.

"What are you doing here?" Jeremy demanded.

"See?" Sterling said to the ship's doctor.

"Shh." Doctor Van Liet held a finger to his lips. "You're on."

"Isn't this cozy," the young doctor snarked. "Anyway, although I recommend a cholecystectomy, the surgeon is not available. He just finished an emergency procedure and is spent. The earliest we could do it is tomorrow morning. I'd like to give you another shot of morphine to get you through the night..."

"I'll stay," Sterling offered.

"Like hell you will," Jeremy shot back.

"Out, both of you." The young doctor pointed at the door.

Jeremy crossed his arms and spread his feet, assuming the position of an immovable tree trunk.

"That's my fault," the ship's doctor admitted. "I brought them together. My only concern is Stephanie, and this man is better for her."

"What?" Jeremy nearly shouted.

"Doc," Stephanie said in a weak voice. Her face pinched with a wave of pain.

Miriam took her hand. "Hang on to me, sister." She was fascinated by the relations, interactions, and posturing. It was like being thrust into the middle of a soap opera, and Stephanie was in the middle of it, suffering. She scanned the many faces in the small room. The E.R. doctor and Sterling were the only two focused on the patient.

Stephanie had her eyes pinched shut as she fought off tears of pain and grief.

Miriam leaned close to her ear and whispered, "Oh, that such men fight over you. An inauspicious honor."

Stephanie snorted. "Doc, you were saying something about a shot of morphine?"

"I want you to understand this will be your last shot unless the pain continues. I don't want you too accustomed to being pain-free. That's not what life is all about, is it?"

"I understand, although I can't be trusted to make this decision. I'm in too much pain and will do or say anything to get it relieved."

"That's the most intelligent thing I've ever heard a patient say in response to more or less morphine. Who do you want to make that decision for you?"

"Please, no, Doc," Stephanie pleaded. "I don't want to make an emotional decision. My lawyer, with advice from my insurance agent. Sorry, Jeremy, but if anything goes wrong, I'll need legal counsel. I think. I'm in pain. I'm not loopy."

"You're plenty clear-headed," Sterling said. He resisted the urge to stare at Jeremy as a sign of dominance. He didn't have to hit the man. Stephanie's words were a blow enough to Jeremy's ego.

The muscles stood out on Jeremy's cheeks from clenching his jaw.

Sterling took morbid pleasure in what he could see using his peripheral vision, but he pulled up short in his mental victory lap seeing Stephanie in pain. It was starting to cause him physical anguish because he felt helpless.

He looked at Miriam. "Morphine?"

"I don't see why not. It's covered. Immediate treatment of symptoms is covered. Tests and follow-ons... Never mind. We can talk about it later." She looked at the E.R. doctor. "Are you recommending a gallbladder removal?"

"Yes," he replied.

"There has to be other options. What if there's no fever?"

"There can still be complications. The ultrasound showed stones. The CT scan didn't see them, so that tells me they're not calcified. She might be able to live with them if they don't get any worse. Stick to a fat-free diet and you might be able to weather this all the way until Stephanie gets home. If you don't have the surgery within four days, then we recommend you get it within three months."

"I'll take that option," Stephanie said. "I can go fat-free between now and then. Take me back to the ship!"

Sterling shook his head. He pointed to the Y-connector where the doctor would inject the pain reliever.

"I'll be right back. No one is to add any more stress to her life. Do you understand me?" He looked at Jeremy first, who ignored him, and then to Sterling, who nodded slowly.

The doctor disappeared. Sterling rested his hand on Stephanie's leg while Miriam held her hand but watched everyone in the room, rapidly switching from one to another to another like she was watching a mixed couples tennis match.

Jeremy resorted to what he was best at—being the life of the party. "How about the renaming of Denali to Mount McKinley, huh? Didn't that come as a complete surprise. Glaciers and all. Nothing is safe from the government eye."

Miriam wasn't sure what to make of Jeremy's diatribe.

An orderly appeared. "I'm moving the patient to her room." He looked at the crowd gathered around her. "I don't think you can come. There's not enough room."

"We're all coming," Jeremy stated. "It's how it's going to be."

"We won't fit in the elevator," the orderly explained.

"Room number?" Jeremy asked. "I'll take the stairs."

"Room Six-Twelve."

"Got it." Jeremy pushed past the others to get to the corridor. He stopped when he was close to Sterling, to glare at him and show his hostility in a way that would be unmistakable.

Sterling didn't need the reminder.

Once Jeremy was gone, Miriam had to ask. "What's his problem?"

Doctor Van Liet jumped into the fray. "You are looking at the only woman in cruise history to bring two men on board in this reverse harem conflagration."

"Reverse harem? Sounds like my type of cruise," Miriam replied. She leaned over Stephanie. "You brought two men on one cruise? Is it turning out how you thought?"

Stephanie shook her head. "I didn't plan any of this. If I had, then I need a shrink and not the ship's doc, no disrespect intended."

"None taken," Van Liet replied with his hands up. The E.R. doc returned with a syringe. He didn't waste any time having the nurse flush the IV line and emptying the morphine into the line. She immediately flushed the line afterward and restored the IV.

Stephanie's relief was almost instantaneous. Her face relaxed and her features smoothed.

"You can take her to her room," the doctor said and tucked her file into a slot at the foot of the bed. "I don't think any of you should go with her. None." He blocked the way as the orderly moved the bed, rolling it down the corridor and away from the insurance agent, one of two boyfriends, and a ship's doctor. "I've never seen anything like this."

He shook his head and walked away.

Miriam was first to concede. "Thank you for your help, kind sir." She smiled at him with her best look, turning slightly to show her figure.

The E.R. doctor swallowed. "We could go over some nuances with how these procedures are billed. Besides you lot, we're not too busy." He gestured for her to join him. Miriam walked away, only to find Jeremy waiting down the hallway.

Jeremy watched her intently, all the way to her heels and back.

Sterling stared blankly at the doorway through which the bed had disappeared. The ship's doctor followed slowly. He'd have to find a ride back to the ship and didn't have a phone with him. He headed for the reception desk.

Jeremy pushed Sterling. "You need to get the hell out of here."

Sterling looked around. It was just them. No one else was in sight.

"I don't. You might have been good for her, just until you weren't. You two aren't going to last, and I suggest you're already done. I'll pick up the pieces of the joy ride you took her on. Unlike you, I love her."

"How much do I love thee who is so lovely as a tree, blah, blah, blah. Are we going to get into a who-loves-her-more contest?"

Sterling shook his head. "What we think doesn't matter. All that matters is what Stephanie thinks and wants."

"Ha! She's already chosen, because she's here with me. You're outta here!" Jeremy made the baseball umpire motion for an out, jerking his thumb over his shoulder.

"Very mature. I'm leaving. I have a plane ticket out of Sydney tomorrow. You shouldn't go gambling when Stephanie is in pain. Show her a little consideration. And making eyes at the insurance agent across Steph's bed? That's as low-class as anyone can be. Congratulations. You're a bottom feeder."

"Who has the girl, smart guy?"

Sterling spread his arms wide. "Looks like neither of us."

Jeremy gave him the finger, and then moved closer until his outstretched arm with middle digit standing tall was inches from Sterling's face.

"Exactly what I'd expect from you. If you'll excuse me, I need to pack." Sterling backed carefully into the corridor. He didn't trust that Jeremy wouldn't attack him. The man was purple with rage but fighting it. Without Stephanie to observe, he might do something he wouldn't otherwise.

Sterling walked away once he was in public again. Doctor Van Liet was waiting for him.

"Thanks, Doc," Sterling told him.

"You're welcome. I've cleared it. You can go up and see her."

"What are you doing?" Sterling was in no mood for games. The last thing he wanted was to make Steph angry. Jeremy was in a perpetual state of high tension. He wished the man would have a heart attack so they could be done with him.

"I'm saving both your lives." The doctor shook Sterling's hand. "I have a taxi to catch. Go to her. Six-Twelve."

Jeremy appeared. "What are you doing?" He glared at both men.

"The insurance agent is available to discuss coverage, including shortfalls. You should probably talk with her. She's down there, in the breakroom." The doctor pointed the way.

Jeremy looked skeptical. "Yeah. We need to get that sorted out. I'll take care of it."

Once he was gone, Sterling mumbled, "Pathetic. Thanks, Doc. See you back on the ship. Maybe not. I already took my stuff off. I'll be going home."

"But not in the clinic. On deck, where normal people congregate."

"Normal people!" Sterling laughed while inching toward the exit from the E.R. "Does any of this look normal?"

The doctor gestured with his head. It was time for both of them to go.

"I won't forget this, Doc." Sterling rushed away.

# CHAPTER THIRTEEN – THE DOGS

STERLING WALKED PAST THE elevators before turning around to make sure Jeremy wasn't watching. He punched the button and waited. A car was available almost immediately. He jumped inside and pressed the button for the sixth floor.

The elevator stopped at the next floor. Two nurses and an orderly squeezed inside with a patient in a wheelchair. The old man moaned and groaned. One nurse kneeled beside him, encouraging him to relax. They rode up two floors and hurried off.

Sterling exited on the next floor. Room 612 was nearby. He peeked in to find it darkened. There were two beds, but one was empty. He eased inside and checked to make sure the person there was who he expected. Stephanie had been hooked up to a cardiac monitor. Her IV bag had been changed.

She looked to be as sick as Sterling thought she was. Three years of seeing her nearly every day, he knew what she looked like before opening his eyes. When he saw her on the ship, he knew instantly that she wasn't healthy.

In bed, lightly sleeping, she looked far better, despite the diagnostics monitoring her every vital.

He lifted a chair and moved it close to the bed, taking care not to make any noise. Sterling sat next to her and held her hand.

He had a million things he wanted to tell her, but he didn't say them. It all boiled down to one thing.

"I love you, Steph," he whispered.

"I love you, too, Sterling," she whispered back.

He wasn't sure he'd heard anything. Her eyes were closed, and she was breathing slowly and rhythmically.

It was what he wanted to hear. He imagined it.

He rested his forehead on their hands.

"Give me time to fix this," Stephanie mumbled.

He lifted his head to find her watching him. Her breathing hadn't changed. Morphine. Keeping her calm.

"Let the doctors fix it," Sterling pleaded. "Nothing you can do about a bum gallbladder."

"That's not what I'm talking about, silly."

"Tell me what you want, and we'll talk about it, compromise, and get a dog."

"You pronounced the word 'cat' funny." She licked her lips and relaxed back into the pillow. She was soon fast asleep once more.

Sterling wondered if he had imagined the conversation. He rested his head on his hands again and stayed that way for a long time, until someone touched his shoulder. He looked up to find a male nurse tapping his watch.

"Time to go. Visiting hours are over."

"When can I come back tomorrow?"

"Eight in the morning," the nurse told him.

He thanked the man. Sterling bent over to kiss Stephanie on her forehead before leaving her alone. He felt much better. He thought for a moment, and then he called the airline to change his plane ticket. He needed to get a hotel room close to the hospital for when he left the ship this very night. His cruise had come to an end.

He'd be here for her through her surgery and recovery. Then they'd fly home together. He assumed Jeremy wouldn't bother sticking around and would continue through the rest of the Pacific.

---

"JOHN." MIRIAM ROLLED THE name over her tongue. "Doctor John. Wasn't that a singer from the sixties?"

"That hurts me at a whole new level. My parents weren't even born back then, but yes, you're not the first to make that joke."

"But I am the cutest."

He shook his head. "My first crush. We were five."

An alarm rang, more of an attention-getter than a klaxon. The hospital wasn't on fire, but a new patient had arrived, and it was all hands on deck. "Back to work," he said and held out his hand.

She stood, and they shook. She gave him her business card. "Call me when you're free. If not tonight, tomorrow. It's still the weekend."

"No guarantee for tonight. I'll call tomorrow when I get off. Maybe we can do dinner or something. I know a good place."

She laughed. "It's Sydney. There are hundreds of good places."

"I was trying to look worldly. Gotta run. I'll call." He rushed into the hallway and nearly ran face-first into the man who had been in the room with one of the patients. "You can't be back here."

"I need to talk with Miriam."

"Not here you don't."

"I was just leaving," Miriam said from behind him. When she saw who it was, her face fell. "On second thought." She returned to the staff breakroom.

"I want to talk to you about Stephanie's coverage," Jeremy stated with conviction.

"No medical power of attorney and no relation, there's nothing I can tell you. I'm sorry."

"Security!" the doctor called down the corridor.

"Fine. I'll wait for you outside," Jeremy called. He turned around and walked toward the door.

The doctor stalled until he was gone and then stuck his head into the breakroom. "Take as long as you want and get security to escort you out." He ran off before she could reply.

Jeremy was a fit man who was fairly good-looking, but he had rubbed Miriam the wrong way. She might have believed in a good enemies-to-lovers romance, but not in this case. She didn't want to have anything to do with him.

Miriam went to the nurse's station. "When does the good Doctor John get off in the morning?"

"His shift ends at eight. Do you have something in mind for the most eligible doctor on shift?"

"How many doctors do you have on shift?"

"One, with one on call."

The nurses laughed.

"See you in the A.M.," Miriam promised. She stopped by the security guard standing at the door.

"There might be a creepy stalker out there. Would you be so kind as to escort me to a taxi?"

"Sure, little miss. Will I need a gun? Because I don't have one. No one in Oz does."

She smiled and shook her head. "Probably not."

Before he opened the door, paramedics rushed by with a blood-covered patient. "He's in V-fib," one stated loudly before they disappeared around the corner. A new alarm sounded in the E.R.

"I hate seeing that, but he's in the right place. If he can be fixed, they'll do it."

"Fixed. Like he's broken?" Miriam wondered.

"We get the most broken, and they show up at the worst of times. Come on, lil miss. We'll get you safely to your cab."

The security guard left the emergency room area, stopping to look around before continuing. Miriam stayed close, between the guard and the wall. There was a taxi stand outside. Instead of the less expensive Uber, she went with the immediate option of a cab. Once she was in and underway, the security guard returned to the E.R.

---

CHIP WOKE UP FROM a fitful sleep earlier than he wanted. He'd made a dog's breakfast of their anniversary by being the right surgeon at the right time. He found himself to be helpless through it all.

Nyla said she wasn't angry and that she had enjoyed the opera, despite having to attend solo. She'd found the couples on either side of her to be delightful. That was the word she used. She was being kind, but then again, she found new friends wherever she went. He wouldn't put it past her to already have plans with them for next weekend.

Time off. When was the last time he had a complete weekend free? The previous weekend when they had nothing planned. Now, he was going in both days. His life was never predictable.

Or as Bethany liked to say, "Routine."

He left Nyla sleeping because it was still early and she'd waited up for him. He had joined her for a quick glass of wine, although he didn't drink his, and then they went to sleep. Chip was exhausted.

Sleep had not been restful, but it was good enough. After a cup of coffee and the travel to the hospital, he'd feel like a new man and be ready to tackle that cholecystectomy. That procedure was quick. Isolate the gallbladder from the liver and remove it. The invasive nature of the surgery was limited because it would be done laparoscopically.

A surgery he could probably perform in his sleep.

He showered, dressed, and almost walked out without taking a garment bag. He returned to their walk-in closet and removed one from a suit. He rolled it up and tucked it under his arm.

Second time leaving the house was successful. He had everything he needed. Chip planned on making quick work of the tourist's gallbladder, but once surgery started, the clock stopped. It would take as long as it needed to take. The team understood that and worked with the same frame of mind.

It took forty minutes to drive himself to the hospital because it was Sunday and traffic was light. A normal day could take an hour to an hour and a half, while public transport, including the ferry, never took longer than an hour.

He parked in the small lot reserved for doctors. He threw yesterday's scrubs, the ones he wore home, into the laundry bin. He stopped by his locker to carefully put his dinner suit into the garment bag. He brushed it with his hands. It was a sharp outfit. They'd paid good money for it, but wearing a cheap dinner suit would never do, not for the events they attended and the aspirations he had.

Chip didn't network to move up. He moved up because he was competent, confident, and published his findings as often as it took to facilitate conversations that would lead to better healthcare, whether systemically or individually.

In his office, he found the digital file on one Stephanie Trent, the tourist from the cruise ship. She was upstairs. He studied the file and found nothing alarming. On the face of it, removal of the gallbladder seemed prudent. He'd see what the patient had to say and how she was feeling after a night's rest.

Chip headed upstairs to Room 612, where he found the patient watching television.

"Anything good on?" he asked.

"I don't recognize any of these shows," she replied. "Are you the surgeon?"

"Chip McClure, at your service." He held up his badge as confirmation. "At least that's what this card says. It has my picture, too. How are you feeling?"

"I think the morphine has worn off, and I don't feel any pain."

Chip checked her abdomen, tapping in the upper right quadrant.

Stephanie shrugged. "Did you guys give me something else? Sonic screwdriver to break the rocks?"

"I'm pretty sure we don't have one of those, but if we did, we would have happily taken care of those stones with it."

He thumped her abdomen until he was sure she was pain-free. "Let's get you up and about. If you're going to walk out of here, we need to make sure you can walk." Chip left to find a nurse to escort Stephanie.

He waved to nurses as he passed. He'd been at the hospital for a lot of years and despite his best efforts, Chip didn't know the entire nursing staff. Turnover wasn't that great. There were a lot of older faces that he recognized, but he didn't know their names. He couldn't do anything about that now besides greet them and try to see the names on their badges.

Chip used the computer at the nurse's station to order the test and let those on shift know. He returned to Stephanie's room to find a man there.

"G'day. I'm Chip." He offered his hand to the man.

"Sterling. Sterling Bower."

"Sterling, like in silver. My twenty-fifth wedding anniversary was yesterday."

"Congratulations. Did you do anything special?" Sterling was making small talk, programmed like he'd trained to do it but his heart wasn't in it. He kept glancing at Stephanie, holding her hand throughout.

"Enough about me. What do you do for a living besides dote on my patient?"

Sterling smiled. It wasn't a smile in response to the observation but for the woman in the bed. It was exactly what Chip saw it to be.

"Lawyer, but please don't hold that against me."

"A lawyer, a doctor, and a patient in the same room. I sense a malpractice suit, and I haven't even operated."

"Did someone say malpractice?" Miriam stood in the doorway.

"Miriam," Sterling said.

"I think I should know you," Stephanie said.

"Last night. You were out of it. I'm Miriam Kiryakova, Unified International Healthcare. I'm your insurance liaison in this region. I don't usually do office calls, but your case stood out. What's the prognosis, Doc?"

"You can call me Chip." He looked to Stephanie for approval, although she would have already given written consent for the insurance company to see everything related to her treatment. She nodded because she understood. Her eyes were clear with normal pupils. They had not given her any more pain-management medications. "I've ordered another ultrasound because Stephanie's condition seemed to have vastly improved. I see no jaundice. There's no tenderness. There's no fever. Although these things don't generally tend to heal themselves, they're not always as bad as temporary pain may indicate."

Sterling chewed over what Chip had told him.

Miriam's brow furrowed. "Yesterday, you looked like imminent death. Today, you look fine."

"I didn't look like imminent death," Stephanie argued. "Although I may have felt like it."

"I never discount a patient's feelings. They know themselves far better than I do."

"That's refreshing," Miriam said. "Too many times, a woman's complaints aren't taken seriously."

"Not in my office." Chip also trusted his gut. People didn't come to see him unless they'd already been vetted. He believed in dispassionate numbers that came from quality diagnostics, appropriate for the malady. That's what he used to make decisions.

Sometimes, the data didn't support how the patient felt. Too often, there was nothing. That's when the doctor had to dig deeper into his bag of tricks, sometimes determine what was wrong through finding things that weren't there when they should have been.

Non-calcified stones in the gallbladder. Were they better or worse? The patient was having no problems, but that was only for the moment.

An orderly appeared. "Ultrasound?" she asked, looking at Doctor McClure.

He pointed at the person in the bed.

"Of course. My first day," she said. She moved in the most bubbly way. The vigor of youth in their new job. "Let's get you to the ultrasound where they can take a right proper look inside that glorious body of yours." She shifted the IV to the hook on the bed. She looked at the ECG lines heading under Stephanie's gown and to a rack next to the wall.

"We can unhook that," Chip said. "I'll take care of it."

The orderly looked disappointed.

"Nurse?" Chip called down the corridor. It was his way of taking care of it. Get the person responsible and let them recover their equipment and appropriately document what was done and when.

The nurse appeared, the one he'd seen when he ordered the test. "I'm sorry. I didn't get your name."

"Sakira Rahim," she replied. "I should have confirmed with you earlier that you'd need the ECG removed. I'm sorry."

"Was there any reason to keep the ECG attached? Any alarms?"

"Nothing," Sakira replied. "Heart beats strong like a horse." She started low and worked her way up. Most had their own methodology for attaching and detaching the leads. Clockwise, big to small, left to right, up and down. Each one needed to be in the correct spot to measure everything from the electrical impulses within the heart to the size of the heart's chambers and the blood flow throughout the body. The ECG could also trigger an alarm at the nurse's station if the body started to shut down. The heart almost always reacted poorly to a body that was dying.

The orderly watched everything the nurse was doing. She asked questions, maybe too many, maybe not. But Nurse Rahim was patient, being a good role model. Chip decided that he didn't need to be there. There was other work he could do while waiting for the results from the ultrasound.

"If you'll excuse me." He bowed his head. "I have some paperwork to do before the results of your test come through."

Miriam followed Chip into the corridor. "We're approved for emergency surgery," she told him. "If it's needed. Your call, of course."

"Thanks." Chip didn't want to pre-judge. The old adage of 'don't operate on people who don't need to be operated on' bounced through his mind. "We'll see what the tests show, and I'll get with the patient, with Stephanie, and see what she wants."

"I like working with you, Chip. You're a straightshooter. No nonsense. No wasted motion."

"There's too much to do to waste what little time we have."

"Hey. I missed you last night," a familiar voice said.

"Oh, God." Miriam ducked into the nearest room—Stephanie's—to hide, but that wouldn't work since that's where Jeremy was going.

"Doc," Jeremy said by way of a greeting as he hurried past.

Chip thought about returning to the room for the inevitable soap opera that was going to unfold. The morbid curiosity of it drew him a step toward the door until he caught himself. "Get a grip!" He hurried toward the elevators before he changed his mind again.

# CHAPTER FOURTEEN – CONFLICT

"WHAT THE HELL ARE you doing here?" Jeremy snarled the instant he saw Sterling. "I thought you were leaving. What will the bar think of your ethics lapse?"

It was a hollow threat. Jeremy held no sway over the Iowa bar, the state licensing body for lawyers.

"I decided to stay." Sterling smiled. He was starting to enjoy getting under Jeremy's skin.

"Excuse us." Nurse Rahim motioned for Jeremy to stop blocking the door. Miriam eased in beside the orderly, hoping to make her escape while being half-hidden behind the bed.

Stephanie watched him with a cold stare. He hadn't bothered to check on her. She was already moving on as soon as the cruise was over, but she thought about moving on before then. Crisis was a window into one's soul. She was old enough that for-better-or-worse meant a great deal.

Jeremy was proving that the for-worse part wasn't his forté.

Sterling, on the other hand. She reached for him as they wheeled her out. She dutifully ignored Jeremy.

"Wait!" he shrieked. "Where are you going?"

"Ultrasound." Sakira gestured for him to move, but he had a grip on the bed's rail.

"She just had one of those last night," Jeremy replied.

"Things change. What? That's what the new test will confirm. Last night was a baseline. Even someone of your intellect can understand that. Please let go."

"Stephanie," he pleaded.

"Let go," Steph told him. She meant far more than just the grip he had on her bed.

Jeremy took a second before complying. He looked up. "Miriam." He tipped his head to her. She helped the orderly push the bed, even though she was dressed up. It was almost eight in the morning, and they'd allowed visitors in early, so she stopped by. But someone she did want to see would be off shift momentarily.

"Gotta run," she said without making eye contact with Jeremy. In the corridor, she let go of the bed and told Stephanie, "You look great. Good luck with your test." She went the other way, opting to take the steps instead of the elevator, make it less likely that Jeremy would follow her.

But he was occupied, if the shouting from the room was any testament.

"I'm gonna kick your ass!"

Miriam covered her ears and ran.

---

STERLING STOOD HIS GROUND, even though there were only the two of them.

Jeremy made fists and raised them. He appeared to have every intent to start punching. "You think she's going with you?"

"You'll have to ask her. I've left the ship. I'm flying out of Sydney and going back home. It's all you. Be the ball."

"What do you mean, be the ball?" Jeremy lowered his fists.

"It's a nineteen-eighties movie reference. I thought you were cultured. I guess not."

"More cultured than you," Jeremy countered.

"Of course. I'll be leaving now." Sterling took the opportunity to rush past Jeremy and into the corridor. He slid sideways down the wall because he didn't want that man to get behind him, but he didn't want to walk backwards down a busy corridor of patients and nurses.

But Jeremy never followed. He stayed in Stephanie's room. Sterling couldn't fathom the reason.

He had changed his plane reservation and his hotel reservation for the three days it would take before Stephanie could travel after gallbladder surgery. If she didn't require surgery, then he could sweep her off the ship sooner.

He might have been presumptuous in buying her a ticket on the flight with him. He wanted to close this chapter and start a new one. He also didn't know what to do about Jeremy. Stephanie didn't know what to do with him either. He was extremely competitive. How would he treat Steph when they were alone? Could she extricate herself from that situation without incurring his wrath?

The challenges were many, but he knew there was one thing that mattered first. The doctor needed to figure out what was going on inside Stephanie's abdomen and treat it. He hated seeing her in pain, but she was getting the medical attention she needed.

It could have been brought on by stress, but reality said that it was exacerbated by stress. What was the underlying cause?

He hoped the ultrasound would give the doctor the answers he sought, the answers they were all looking for.

---

THE NOTIFICATION POPPED UP on Chip's computer that the ultrasound results were in. He checked them over to find that there was a small change from the previous day's results. The stones measured at half a millimeter smaller. It could have been a change of angle, but the bottom line was that the surgery was no longer an emergency.

He stood ready to operate, but time was no longer the limiting factor.

Chip headed upstairs to meet with Stephanie.

Her room had transformed in the past ninety minutes. Flowers covered every horizontal surface. There were even three mylar balloons. One encouraged her to get well and the other two professed love.

Chip wondered which of Stephanie's suitors had pulled out all stops to win her over. His money was on the rude one. The man wasn't that young, but he was younger than Chip by a good measure and had yet to learn that buying favors never worked.

"Stephanie?" Chip called from the doorway, leaning around the egregious displays.

"Doctor." She waved him in.

"Your gallstones are still present, but there is no swelling of the gallbladder wall. That could account for your feeling better. I don't think we *have* to operate anymore as an emergency, but we can. There's still an issue with your gallbladder, and I expect it'll have to come out eventually to forestall worse complications."

"I don't need the surgery? So, I can go..."

"No, you don't need surgery, *not right now*," Chip clarified, already second-guessing whether he should have been more persistent about the gallbladder removal. The unvarnished truth created a dilemma where the patient would cause more problems for themselves. "And that's the most I can say. What are you going to do?"

"I have to go back to the ship to collect my things. I'd like to go to Vietnam at some stage to see where my dad had been, but maybe once I'm feeling myself again..."

"And I'm going to show it to her," Jeremy said from behind a massive vase of flowers.

Doctor John from the E.R. and Miriam showed up at Stephanie's room. Miriam grunted incoherently when she saw the flower madness within.

"Miriam," Jeremy said while holding onto Stephanie's arm.

Doctor John stepped forward. "G'day, mate. Call me John." He offered his hand as if they were meeting for the first time and not that he'd threatened to call security on Jeremy the night before.

Jeremy crossed his arms.

Miriam had to maneuver through the room to get to Stephanie. She put the bed between her and Jeremy while John stood in the way.

"What did the test show?" she asked.

"That I don't need surgery, at least not right now," Stephanie said in a normal voice. Her face wasn't pinched from pain, and her color was good.

"No emergency surgery?" Miriam clarified.

"No."

Miriam tapped away on her phone, frowning.

"What?" Stephanie looked concerned.

"Well, if it's not emergency surgery, then it's elective and your insurance won't cover it."

"Whew, that's a relief, because I have no intention of having surgery that I don't need, but I'll take required surgery, for reference. Not here, anyway. No disrespect to the staff at Westpark. There are some things that are better done in the comfort of one's own home." Stephanie sounded confident as she proclaimed her plan for the future.

"Thank you for understanding, Stephanie, and I wish you the best. I'm pretty sure we'll cover most of what you've gone through. Leave it to me and I'll send you an email to the address in the account." Miriam patted Stephanie's arm with the relief they both felt.

"Works for me. I want to see someone about what it'll take to get discharged. I need to get my stuff from the ship."

"What?" This time, it was Jeremy who was confused. "We're going to Vietnam."

"No. *We* are not. Weren't you listening? I'm going to Vietnam, but not right now. I'm going home. This whole thing was a mistake, but I'm not going to abandon my stuff. Back to the ship to pack and disembark."

Jeremy shrugged. "If that's what you want. You looked forward to seeing Vietnam. There's no sense in diving off now when you're so close and you're feeling better."

"So close to this gallbladder going sideways. I'd prefer not to be at sea when it does."

"But being on an airplane is okay?" Jeremy argued.

"Being on an airplane soon when I feel okay. Every flight gets me that much closer to home. That's where I want to be."

Jeremy's lip twitched as he wrestled with his anger and the competition that marked every aspect of his life. He was losing, and there wasn't much he could do about it.

"Then that's what we'll do. Get you back to the ship and I'll bring you home."

"Not you, no. Continue your cruise and enjoy your time in the casino and wherever else you want to be." Stephanie raised her head. "We're done, Jeremy."

Miriam covered her face when she wanted to cheer for Stephanie and give her a hug. Stephanie had confronted Jeremy in front of other people when some things were best done in private.

If you feel safe. If not, then definitely in public.

"I'll help you pack, but I don't want to see you go."

"We'll be off, then," Miriam blurted. She grabbed John's arm as she hurried past. Even though Stephanie appeared to want them there, for moral support or some other reason, it was too awkward.

"Miriam," Jeremy called after her, but she ignored him.

John held her hand as they walked to the elevators. "You know, the hand is one of the dirtiest places on the human body. The mouth is next."

Miriam stared while they waited for the next car. "You don't date much, do you?"

"Too busy with med school, interning, and everything else that goes into being a world-class doctor. Why do you ask?"

"No reason. It was a wild guess."

---

STERLING WAITED AT THE hotel, like he and Stephanie had agreed, as much as it grated on his very soul. She didn't want to have surgery, but she'd call him when she was certain. He had reservations for three days, and their plane tickets were for the day they'd check out of the hotel.

If she did have surgery, then he'd be there with her every step of the way, ready to fly as soon as she was able.

He paced in his room, replaying every interaction, every look, every word. Jeremy's face kept appearing. The hard question he had to face was, could he put that man behind him? Stephanie had seen something in him, and then the spark faded. That had to be good enough. She was moving on by moving back to Sterling.

*Find solace in her eyes and kind words,* he counseled himself. It was easy to tell yourself to do something or, even harder, to stop doing something, but it was much more difficult to put into practice. Yet, if Sterling was going to live the life he wanted with the woman he loved, then that's exactly what he had to do.

He continued to pace while the phone sat there, not ringing.

# CHAPTER FIFTEEN – ESCAPE

"THAT'S IT. YOU'RE CLEARED to go." Stephanie was in a wheelchair because that was hospital policy. She was spry and feeling good, better than she had the whole trip so far. She'd gotten plenty of sleep, finally.

The only thing causing her stress at the moment was Jeremy, but he wasn't being his usual self. He was far quieter than normal. She didn't know what to make of that since he was never quiet for very long. She expected to get an earful once they were alone.

Outside, there was a line of taxis waiting for their next customer. They flagged the first vehicle and climbed in.

Jeremy stayed silent.

Stephanie didn't encourage him. The taxi headed to the harbor where the big cruise liner was berthed.

Jeremy paid with his card, and they got out. Stephanie walked slowly because she didn't want to enrage the gallbladder gods. She only wanted to get her luggage and have a purser carry it to the gangway so she could leave. In between, she'd find time to call Sterling. She felt a fool for all of it.

The buffoon had showed her an exciting life, yet she'd ignored the red flags he kept tossing in his wake.

Not anymore.

They walked up the gangplank. Stephanie looked for her passenger card but couldn't find it.

Jeremy flashed both his and hers.

"I'll take that," she told him, but he shoved both cards into his pocket.

He shook his head and kept walking. "You don't need it to get off the ship. I'd like a memento of our trip, as bad as it's turning out. If I want to be a better man, I have to learn from my failures. At least, that's what my heart is telling me."

She listened, but it sounded too contrived. Just like the rainforest of flowers he'd had delivered to her room, it didn't come across as sincere. How much money had he wasted on such an extravagant display?

They headed toward their room, but Jeremy perked up as if he heard something. "Lunch is being served. One last meal together?" He looked at her with pleading eyes. She was nothing if not empathetic. She had just delivered hard news in the hardest way. She didn't see the harm.

They went to the buffet since the dining room was closed while they were in port. The options were limited.

He took his time and spoke of inane things. There was no reminiscing, just a view of a world he had not yet seen but would. Petra in Jordan. The Burj Khalifa in Dubai. The Parthenon in Athens. Dai Butsu in Japan. Mount Fuji, too.

The state of a nation long away and a world worth living in, where people could go about their lives without fear.

When they finally finished, they strolled past a champagne bar, where Jeremy ordered two. He kept talking about the most innocuous of things. They toasted the good weather. It was easy to agree on something like that. Summer down under with winter back home.

Stephanie excused herself to go to the bathroom so she could have a few minutes of privacy. She decided to text Sterling instead of calling him because she didn't want to set Jeremy off.

He was acting weird, most unlike himself. Distant and disengaged.

*We're headed to the room now. Ten minutes to pack and then to the dock. I'll take a taxi to the hotel. I look forward to seeing you. xoxoxo*

She returned to find Jeremy close to the bathroom door. He nodded politely, and they walked slowly to the cabin.

Stephanie rushed, but Jeremy's movements were more deliberate. He was in her way or moving things back and forth under a pretense of packing more efficiently.

The ship announced that they would be leaving shortly.

"Jeremy! I need to go. Get out of my way."

His demeanor changed instantly. He stood in front of the door with his arms crossed. "You see, now we have a problem. I paid for two for this room; I'm going to get my money's worth. You're not getting off the ship."

"Let's talk about this, because there's no way I'm going to let you kidnap me. No way!" She brandished a lamp like a baseball bat. She hadn't finished packing because of Jeremy's interference. Red lights flashed in front of her eyes. If she didn't get off the ship now, she'd be trapped. Sterling wouldn't be able to help her. Or could he?

She pulled out her phone and started tapping away. Jeremy struck like a cobra, snatching the phone out of her hand. He swung a fist at her but didn't touch her. It was to get her attention.

He deleted what she typed and sent something else.

*Changed my mind. Staying with Jeremy.*

He smashed the phone against the doorframe. He pounded it so hard that it scared Stephanie. His features were wild, unhinged. Jeremy dropped what was left of the phone on the deck. He kicked it away.

"No sense crying about it. You're going to get to see Vietnam, and in between, you'll learn to love me." He spoke evenly, calmly, even though his eyes were wide and his fingers twitched compulsively.

"How do you think that's going to happen? I will fight you with every fiber of my being," Stephanie declared. She had just earned her freedom to make her own choices and wasn't going to give that up.

But her choices hadn't been great lately. Jeremy was one of them. Taking this ill-advised trip was another. It was time to go home and stop pretending to be a world-traveler. Stop pretending to be a daredevil. The thought of home never felt so good as it did right now, but it had moved beyond her control. She sat on the side of the bed, resisting the urge to cry. She kept a tight grip on the lamp.

She was being kidnapped! It was time for her to be strong. The only one who could save her was her.

Stephanie stood. "Move out of the way, Jeremy. I'm leaving, and you can have all my stuff. There's not a damn thing I need here." She grabbed her purse before he could get it. Her passport should have been inside, but it wasn't.

"You planned this."

"I planned the whole trip. I planned everything, except for you to get sick, but now that I see you, I'm not so sure you were as sick as you made out to be. Maybe I can get myself some morphine by playing footsies with the ship's doc. No, I wouldn't do that since I need to be clear-headed." He lifted his chin and looked down his nose at her.

She brandished her lamp, trying to be as menacing as she could, but he only laughed.

"The last thing you are is clear-headed. Kidnapping is a felony, Jeremy. Let me go now and I won't tell anyone."

"I can't do that. We're not at sea yet. Once you've cut the umbilical cord to that piece of trash lawyer, you'll see. We were meant to be together, Steph."

"That's enough. You're acting like the *Silence of the Lambs* guy. Are you going to tell me to put lotion on my skin?" She jumped forward and swung the lamp, but Jeremy was faster. He met her halfway and caught the lamp before she could bring it down on his head. He yanked it out of her hand.

"Don't be that way."

"I'm going to start screaming," Stephanie threatened.

"You won't like what I do if you exercise your vocal cords, so please don't." His tone was ice cold.

She had been afraid of Jeremy before now, but nothing like this. Everything he'd done on this day had been to deny Stephanie the chance to leave. He drew her in and acted non-confrontational until it was too late.

The trap had been sprung, and she was caught.

She flopped onto the bed and hung her head. A spasm launched through her abdomen.

Stephanie gasped and held herself, right below the ribs. "Oh, no," she cried out.

"I'm not falling for that again. You're going to stay right here while I go play poker. I'm feeling lucky." He gestured toward the window. "There's nowhere for you to go." The harbor bridge passed slowly as the ship moved under it and headed toward the open sea.

Jeremy left the room. Outside, he fumbled with the lock. Stephanie wondered where he'd gotten a key to the room, but he did, and the lock clicked into the frame like a deadbolt. She checked the knob, but she couldn't get the lock to disengage.

She was stuck. Stephanie got on her hands and knees to dig under the desk, the last place she'd seen her phone. The screen was shattered, but she had a screen protector that kept it all in place. She tapped it, and it came to life and recognized her. She accessed the messaging app and sent Sterling a new message.

*Jeremy has kidnapped me. Call for help. Gallbladder is acting up once more. Help me!*

*On my way,* Sterling replied.

*Already at sea. Send help.*

*On it. Hang tough. Help is on the way.*

Stephanie stared at the screen. The spiderwebs across the glass made it difficult but not impossible. She was amazed it worked.

She thought, *Play his game*. She deleted the most recent texts and put the phone back on the floor under the desk. She'd have to count on Sterling. She found comfort in that thought, which told her everything she needed to know.

Pain radiated through her entire body, starting from the one place she thought had given her a respite. Stephanie filled a plastic cup and drank it down. She drank a second. She had nothing with her to help. She assumed the phone in the room was disconnected, and it was. The connector from the line into the phone had been mangled.

Jeremy had been planning this for a while. The door lock. The phone. The passport and boarding card.

The flowers were a distraction. A hugely competitive man who was on the verge of losing something he considered important. He hated to lose.

Stephanie didn't see herself as a prize. It was a flight of fancy, her imagination run rampant where she was desirable, but that was something completely different. There was an allure to being the apple in good men's eyes. If only Jeremy had been what he appeared to be.

She went onto their balcony and thought about jumping, but it was too far down to the water, and they were already far out at sea. Depending on the tide, it could sweep her farther out to sea despite her best swimming efforts. The ship moved along at a good clip.

She leaned around to see if others nearby were on their balconies to ask them for help, but there was no one that she could see. "Hello? Can someone help me? I'm trapped in my room. The door lock is broken. Hello?" She cupped her hands around her mouth to shout one way and then the other.

Nothing.

She would have thought more people would be outside, enjoying the view from the privacy of their own stateroom while the ship headed out to sea, but line dancing and other scheduled entertainment had distracted them from enjoying some of the more subtle delights the cruise had to offer.

"Hello?" she shouted once more. Disinterested. Disengaged. Or simply not there. The ship hadn't been full, but there were still plenty of people.

Stephanie was in survival mode. Another weapon. Or gymnastics. She could crawl around to the next balcony.

A wave of pain coursed through her body. It was bad, worse than before. Relief had been, as it turned out, fleeting. She doubled over and then fell to her knees on the balcony. The sea air had a unique smell when mixed with the power of diesel. It wasn't completely unpleasant.

A weapon. If she could stand, she could find something to pummel Jeremy with. If she were to escape, it would take beating Jeremy in a physical contest. He'd be ready for her. She'd have to bide her time, but the only thoughts she had were for the pain raging within her body.

The only problem with being kidnapped was that she couldn't see the doctor. There were more problems than that, but right now, seeing the doctor topped her list.

She should have taken the surgery and never come back to the ship. But it was elective and wouldn't be covered.

How about now? Stephanie argued with herself. She crawled into the room. The non-skid of the balcony deck tore at her knees. The carpet in the stateroom was welcome. She tried to pull herself upright on the bed, but she didn't have enough strength.

She had been strong enough to swing a lamp at Jeremy's head, but now she didn't have the strength to stand. How quick were the issues that plagued her? How terrible the resurgence of pain, which had returned with a vengeful spite that told Stephanie it was her time to suffer.

Her failure would be complete.

For the first time in her life, she felt like she was going to die. She curled up on the floor. The pain didn't subside. It cycled between bad and debilitating. She gasped with each breath, panting until she was lightheaded. She fought for every breath, every second of consciousness. She was afraid that if she closed her eyes, she wouldn't open them again.

She was afraid that Jeremy would return.

And then she was afraid that he wouldn't.

# CHAPTER SIXTEEN – SALVATION?

CHIP LOOKED DOWN AT Roo's daughter. She was asleep in the chair in his room. She had stayed there all night while her father went through the worst of it. He saw the grim reaper and decided it wasn't his time to shake hands.

Roo rested. His body was on the winning side of the fight for life, but it left him exhausted. His obs looked solid, much stronger than when he finished surgery the previous evening. Chip was happy he hadn't died. It wouldn't have been Chip's fault, but Roo could speak to his community about how he could have died but didn't because of a recommended surgery. His daughter could be a modern medicine evangelist, too.

Chip strolled to his car. After three blissful hours catching up on paperwork, narrating surgery notes into the system and closing out files, he was finished, and it wasn't the last minute on Sunday. He still had plenty of day remaining.

He strolled out of the hospital and into the warm midday sun. Chip stopped to take in the heat and a healthy amount of vitamin D. Not too much. He didn't need a sunburn and in this part of the world at this time of year, fifteen minutes was all it would take.

He was pastier than most since he saw very little of the sun with his day-to-day duties. Golf was different. He covered up and used copious amounts of sun block. He called Nyla to let her know he was on his way.

It felt good to save a life, even though he also felt guilty about not being able to talk Roo into surgery sooner. Sometimes, the cards didn't fall your way. He thought about the American, Stephanie, and the menagerie of characters surrounding her. He chuckled. There's no way that wasn't stressful.

Miriam had been there at the beginning and helped Stephanie, but the insurance people had their own agenda. Having them involved up front sometimes led to bad decisions based on what was covered versus what was needed. He was convinced that Stephanie needed surgery, but he couldn't strong-arm her into getting it. She felt fine when she left the hospital, but for how long? She'd eventually go under the knife.

Maybe it was better for her back in America. As long as the stones didn't migrate out of her gallbladder and cause problems by blocking her bile duct. That would be bad. Chip had made sure his notes were comprehensive since he expected the next doctor would see them. If it was an emergency, the doctor would need the best information as quickly as possible. If it wasn't, a good record would help the next surgeon by having a complete record.

The drive home was easy enough. Traffic had picked up by midday, but it was still Sunday and nowhere near what was possible on a workday. Traffic jams, accidents, and anger were all too common in big city traffic. That was the norm across the globe. Heavy traffic was never something that brought happiness into anyone's lives.

Chip was no exception. He didn't enjoy driving in it and only did it on rare occasions when he needed the car to haul something or had multiple and random stops between work and home. Sometimes, Nyla would ask him to pick up odds and ends. He'd do it because that's what good husbands did.

Unlike that free-for-all he witnessed between the two men vying for Stephanie's affection. He wondered how that would play out. The soap opera of a doctor's daily life.

*General Hospital* out of the United States was one such soap. It ran five days a week for more than sixty years and was still going strong. People tuned in to see the daily drama.

Chip had to laugh. He saw enough in real life that he didn't need the sensationalized version. They got too much wrong for him to get invested.

---

MIRIAM LEANED IN AS Doctor John kissed her on the cheek. They'd gone to a breakfast place for something light. He had yogurt and granola, stating that he had to maintain his health because the shifts in the E.R. were so grueling. He hadn't managed to get any sleep so far, but the nurses promised him there would be times he could take a nap. He didn't believe it, but he was quickly running out of gas. He summoned an Uber and left Miriam standing on the corner.

She liked him. He'd passed the first date test and had earned a second.

Things were looking up. She headed to the quay to take in the departure of the cruise liner. They seemed to bring her clients. Maybe she'd see something to help Unified International's marketing department in encouraging travelers to get expanded coverage on their healthcare plans when they went overseas.

"What to do now?" she asked herself. She looked around to make sure no one was nearby to judge her for talking to herself.

She was riding solo but not for long. She had high hopes for the new doctor. He was her age, which wasn't that young any longer. She took care of herself so young men were interested, as well as much older men.

She snorted at the incongruity of it all. Miriam was an executive with an important job. Even though there was never going to be complete client satisfaction, she could make their experience with emergency healthcare less painful than it already was.

A coffee shop was nearby, and it wasn't busy. She selected a corner table that was out of the way. She put in her AirPods and started calling her country liaisons, just to check in on them and ask what she could do to help. In her job, that personal touch made all the difference. Insurance was already mostly hands-off and too impersonal.

She would do her part to hold the computer age at bay.

"Makshur, sorry to call on a Sunday, and I'll tell you that I don't need anything. I want to make sure that you're okay. How are you doing?"

she started every conversation the same way. She was a trained extrovert. She was fine having no contact with humanity, but she was good at engaging others. She saw it as a mental chess match. Maneuvering around a verbal board to make sure the conversation went her way. Get them to tell all while she said very little.

It was the game she played.

She sipped her latte while encouraging her liaisons to talk, but not for long. It was Sunday. She excused it by telling them they were too busy during the week to speak casually.

Casual and open. A conversation that made people feel comfortable. She needed her liaisons to be at ease when talking with her. No repercussions for telling the truth as they saw it.

All truth had shades of gray. She was good at seeing that, too. Some called it empathy. Others called it emotional intelligence. She saw it as simple elements of debate. Dissect and examine. Restate and clarify.

In her business, there couldn't be any confusion, even though confusion usually worked to the insurance company's benefit. The more confused providers and patients were, the less had to be paid out. That led to bad reviews on the low end and lawsuits on the high end. She wanted neither.

Clarify up front. Like she'd done with Stephanie. Not an emergency. Stephanie needed a better policy.

Miriam pulled up Stephanie's policy on her phone. She upgraded her policy to the premier version with a couple clicks. She'd set herself a reminder to downgrade the policy back to normal before the balloon payment came due.

Just in case Stephanie ran into problems while visiting other ports. Everywhere except Indonesia. Unified International provided no coverage for services performed in that country. The coverage wasn't perfect, but it was better than being tossed in a foreign jail for not being able to pay.

That was probably an old wives' tale, something to scare people. She couldn't imagine any patient being jailed for their inability to pay their hospital bill. She'd have to check that. It piqued her interest.

---

JEREMY DROPPED HIS TWO jacks on the table where the third was already up. He threw his hands in the air in triumph! His luck was holding. That was five hands out of six. He scooped the chips off the table.

"That's it for me. I have to check on the little lady. She's a bit under the weather. Important safety tip: Don't eat seafood from a food truck that's been in the sun all day."

The group of players nodded knowingly. He waved and took his haul to the cashier.

"Credit or payout," she asked.

"I'll take a payout for now. I'll probably be back, but I might not be. I'll be busy with tours. Something new in every port. What a great cruise! Do you get off the ship much?"

She shook her head. "It's hard work. The best benefit is that we aren't able to spend any of the money we make. Call it forced savings. I share a small room with three other women. The only thing we do in there is sleep. Food is provided. We can't use the guest gym, and our facilities are less than exemplary. Still, it's a way to make some money before I decide what I want to do with my life."

"You have your head on straight, and that means your hand will come up aces. It's not luck. It's good, hard work focused on a singular goal." He gave her the thumbs-up and walked away. He stopped by the hot dog stand and ordered one with chili and fries. He took a seat at one of the few tables for the stand's customers and devoured his impromptu meal.

He wasn't in a hurry. The switch had flipped, and he no longer carried the weight of his concerns on his conscience. He was winning. At everything. He only had to figure out how to win over Stephanie before they disembarked. If he couldn't, he suspected that she'd throw herself overboard. Until then, though, he had a chance.

Jeremy had utmost confidence in himself. He'd win her affection. Go back to the way it was before. He'd describe the exotic things they would do, and then they would go do them. It was his way.

*Live up to your dreams,* he told himself. He finished but sat for a few moments before tossing his trash. He headed for the room, fingers caressing the key in his pocket.

Stephanie would apologize for being obstinate. She would see that he was right. And then they'd go for a walk around the top deck, arm in arm, enjoying the sights and sounds of their ship.

He turned the key slowly so he wouldn't make noise. He yanked the door open and crouched, in case someone was waiting with a club or ready to throw something, but there was no one inside. He checked behind the door before stepping inside.

Stephanie wasn't in the bathroom or on the bed or on the balcony, but the balcony door was open.

Had she thrown herself overboard? No way. He didn't see her having that kind of strength. He took a step inside and saw her on the floor.

"You can get up now. I'm not falling for that." He eased close to her to nudge her with his toe. She was on her side. He backed away and turned on all the lights in the room. She didn't move.

He leaned down, ready to fight her off if she had a weapon, but her skin was flushed. Her hands hung limp and weren't holding anything. He rolled her to her back and lifted her eyelids to see if she would focus on him.

The whites of her eyes were distinctly yellow.

He picked up her limp form and put her into bed. Jeremy covered her up.

"What to do with you?" he asked. "So much for exciting day trips in exotic locations."

He took a sip of water and watched her. She was unconscious with yellow eyes and a fever. What did that mean?

Jeremy checked the balcony, but people were outside on either side. That removed the option of throwing her overboard. No matter. She would never know that was an option. He left the room, carefully locking it before walking down the corridor to a phone on the wall. He dialed the number for the clinic. A nurse answered the phone.

"Jeremy Dissick in Room Six-Twenty-Seven. My girlfriend is ill. I think she passed out. She's Stephanie Trent. That's right. She was taken off on a stretcher in Sydney. Gallbladder but not bad enough to operate. Symptoms? Her eyes are yellow, and she has a fever. How long? I don't know. I wasn't here. When I came back, she was unconscious."

The nurse told him they would be there immediately.

He had been hoping for a different answer, like give her water or make sure she's comfortable. After a moment's reflection, he realized how ridiculous that was. Deep down, he didn't want to lose her. His thoughts of sending her overboard were ill-conceived and short-lived. He wanted to think he could do it out of necessity, but reality suggested something far different. Keeping her in the room until he could win her over was one thing. Killing her was something else completely.

He'd played poker to let her cool off, realize that he was trying to help her. Like calling the doctor. He was still helping her. Where would she be without him?

No. She needed to survive so she could embrace him once more and he could flaunt that in Sterling Bower's face. Only one could win this battle. He wasn't going to share his woman with anyone else. It was that Bower guy. He needed to go.

But he was already gone. He'd left the ship. She had been hurrying to join him. With the last text, he'd be rid of him. No more Sterling Bower. She hadn't joined him in Sydney, and now there was no way for him to contact her.

Victory!

Except the minor fact that she was unconscious. Jeremy hurried to the cabin and unlocked the door. He didn't have to wait long for the ship's doctor.

"What did you do?" Doctor Van Liet snapped.

"I called you to help Stephanie. Your bedside manner, Doc, getting knee-deep where you don't belong? You might want to check that, because you don't want to make me angry."

Jeremy's tone was angry at first but turned cold toward the end. The multiple personalities of one man showed through in a short exchange.

The doctor stopped before entering. "My apologies. May I see her?"

Jeremy nodded and stepped aside.

The doctor hurried in. He checked her eyes. "She's febrile and jaundiced," he stated.

"Febrile?"

"Has a fever. It's the sign of infection we didn't want to see. Jaundice probably means her bile duct is blocked. The stone migrated."

Jeremy threw his hands up. "So, what does all that mean?"

"It means we need to evacuate her off the ship right now or she'll die. She needs the surgery she didn't get, but now it's no longer an option."

The nurse appeared and leaned in the doorway. She'd heard part of the conversation. "Doctor?"

"I'm ordering a medevac." He picked up the room's phone, but it was dead. He called to the nurse. "Order a medevac, soon as you can, for an emergency. Acute cholangitis. Have a surgeon ready to receive her."

Why was the room's phone dead? The doctor didn't have time to think about it more than grumbling about the inefficiency of using the phone down the corridor.

She ran to the phone and called the bridge. The nurse spoke loudly enough for all to hear. "On the orders of Doctor Van Liet, request an emergency medevac via helicopter for acute cholangitis. She'll need surgery. Quick as you can, please. Advise ETA. I'll wait."

The doctor checked Stephanie's pulse and blood pressure, shaking his head with each new piece of information. "How long has she been like this?"

"Don't know. I found her when I returned to the room."

The doctor stared while biting his tongue to keep from unloading on the young man. She needed constant attention so something like this wouldn't progress any longer than necessary. "Say, no more than three hours?" They'd been at sea for five.

"No more than three. That's ballpark." Jeremy was minimally committal.

The ship's doctor was less than amused. "We'll need to move her to the infirmary, where we can give her an IV while we wait for the helicopter."

Jeremy chewed the inside of his lip while contemplating his next move. "There's nothing you can do here?"

"There is nothing I can do except keep her comfortable until the helicopter arrives. Please understand, *she's dying*. She has run out of time."

"That's disconcerting," Jeremy said.

The doctor fought his urge to choke the man. He decided to focus on his patient.

"Forty-five minutes," the breathless nurse announced.

"Stretcher," the doctor ordered.

"Come with me," she told Jeremy. She ran down the corridor. There was a stretcher strapped to the bulkhead on each deck. There was never one far away.

Jeremy jogged after her. She freed it from the wall, and he caught the far end. Together, they walked back to the room. They opened the stretcher and laid it inside the doorway. The doctor and the nurse muscled Stephanie onto the stretcher while Jeremy stood back.

"I'll help carry her," Jeremy offered.

"Just hold the door. We have her," the doctor replied. They continued down the passageway to the freight elevator used exclusively by the staff.

When the nurse punched the button, she looked past the doctor. He turned his head to find Jeremy standing right behind them.

"Wait in your room. We'll call with an update."

"I have to go to the hospital with her."

"No room on the whirlybird, mate," the nurse said, saving the doctor from having to tell him no.

"I'm going." Jeremy allowed no dissent. Van Liet intended to call the bridge in private and tell them under no circumstances was this man to get on that helicopter.

He didn't know exactly what was going on, but none of it was good. A patient that was dying because of the inattention of her so-called boyfriend. The man was a menace. If not actively complicit, then negligent.

There was nothing the good doctor could do about it.

They carried the stretcher into the infirmary, akin to a community urgent care facility, and put the stretcher on the bed. The nurse readied the IV and looked for a new place to insert it since Stephanie had had one in her right arm for an extended period. The nurse picked the left arm, placed a tourniquet in the upper part, found a vein, and swabbed the skin clean. The doctor took a temperature strip from his kit and placed it carefully under the patient's tongue.

He looked at her eyes again while the temperature strip warmed to thirty-nine degrees Celsius, which was a shade over one hundred and two Fahrenheit. The fever had come on quickly, just like the jaundice.

Stephanie was dying, and Doctor Van Liet didn't have to exaggerate or sensationalize. The emergency was real. Three hours in a coma due to acute cholangitis. Forty-five minutes to the helicopter, and then another thirty minutes to get back to the hospital. Surgery prep, assuming there was a surgeon available. She could be in the operating room in under two hours.

The doctor kept checking the clock on the wall. It made it obvious.

"How much time does she have?" Jeremy asked.

It was an innocuous question but one where the doctor was afraid of the answer. "More than two hours. It better be, anyway."

"Why's that?" Jeremy pressed.

"Because that's how long it'll take to get her into surgery."

"What if she doesn't have that long?"

"Then she won't need surgery," the doctor replied without emotion. It was a statement of fact. He needed her to hang on.

He hadn't been as insistent about her getting her gallbladder removed as he should have been. Stones don't go away. He knew that. The surgeon had explained it, allowing Stephanie to decide. Now she suffered the consequences of her decision and a boyfriend who let her suffer for far too long.

She'd have to survive five hours in a coma, while febrile and jaundiced.

The IV delivered fluids, but that wouldn't keep her body from shutting down. Van Liet started an infusion of antibiotics. Toxins and bacteria from the gallbladder, as well as a massive inflammatory response would kill her as surely as a severe heart attack caused by a complete blockage of the left anterior descending artery, infamously called the widow maker. Stephanie had her own widow maker in a blocked bile duct.

"Keep fighting, young lady," Doctor Van Liet told her. Someone had to because Jeremy hadn't said a word to her. The doctor looked up to find Jeremy watching. He wasn't giving the doctor a moment alone to call the bridge. "What's going on?"

"I don't understand. You said she was sick."

"I'm talking between you two. I thought she was going with that other guy. Silver, whatever his name was." The doctor was flustered. Jeremy's look was cold and calculating. He stared at Van Liet without blinking until the doctor looked away. He put his stethoscope in his ears and listened to her heart once more. He didn't need to but couldn't think of anything else to do to kill time.

"Nurse," Doctor Van Liet said to get her attention. "Keep your eye on the patient. I need to fill out some forms so there's no delay taking her back to Sydney." He looked at Jeremy. "We'll need her passport."

"Right here." Jeremy pulled it out of his pocket and held it up. He wouldn't have to go back to the room for it.

"Fine. Thank you. I'll take it."

Jeremy put it back in his pocket. "I'll give it to the authorities myself." He kept his hand in his pocket and made no other moves.

The air in the room grew stale and hot.

"Don't you have forms to fill out?" Jeremy asked.

"Right." Doctor Van Liet retired to his office. He flipped the door shut behind him, but it didn't close. It bounced off Jeremy's foot.

"I'm here if there's anything you need."

"Of course." A bead of sweat rolled down the doctor's forehead and into his eye. A second bead followed. He was on fire, but not from a fever. Anxiety. Stress. Fear. What was this man capable of?

The doctor hadn't found anything untoward from what he could see of Stephanie's body. And Jeremy had called the doctor when he found her. Maybe he was afraid that he'd be accused of abusing her through negligence, even though she was the one who refused the surgery. She was the one who came back to the ship.

The suitcase on the dresser. Mostly packed. She was leaving, and Jeremy stopped her. The doctor hadn't realized he'd seen the suitcase or what it meant. Stress was a killer. Could it be responsible for migrating a stone? The body reacting to perceived and real threats. Never say never.

Doctor Van Liet removed a couple forms from a filing cabinet, neither of which were necessary, but Jeremy didn't know that. The doctor focused on filling in the information and then folded both forms and put them in his pocket.

"Can I see those?"

"Under no circumstances. Are you family?"

"Almost," Jeremy countered.

"You are not. You do not have a medical power of attorney. You have no legal right to see any medical information as it relates to my patient, and it's illegal for me to show it to you. So, no. You shouldn't even be in here, but if I ordered you to leave, you wouldn't go, would you?"

"No." Jeremy shook his head. "Don't bother calling security, either. We don't want to make a fuss in front of Stephanie. She needs her rest."

If it was possible for Jeremy to stall, that's what he was doing, but the helicopter wasn't there yet. The doctor checked the time. Still twenty minutes before the medevac arrived.

The clock seemed to be ticking louder than normal.

The nurse turned the temperature down in the office. She was sweating, too.

Stephanie's skin was starting to change color, turning yellow from the jaundice.

"Stay strong, little lady. It won't be much longer now."

# CHAPTER SEVENTEEN – PARITY

STERLING TRIED TO CALL the ship, but he kept getting cut off. He tried to call Stephanie's phone, but it was off. He managed to get through to the Coast Guard, but all they did was take a report.

He even called Miriam Kiryakova, the insurance representative. She had recognized Jeremy for the lowlife he was. He hoped she could recommend something.

She had no idea what to do besides call the entities he had already called. Then it came to her.

"I have a number for an office of the cruise line. It's right here in Sydney." She gave it to him.

"I'll call them and see if they can contact the ship. I'm worried, Miriam. I'll call you back with what they tell me."

She didn't need him to call her, except through the fascination of watching a slow-motion trainwreck. She wanted to know how everything turned out. Stephanie kidnapped?

Could she have predicted it? No one could have.

Sterling called the cruise liner's office and was redirected to an answering machine. The ship was gone and so were the local staff. Sterling left a message anyway. "My girlfriend is on the ship. She's been kidnapped. We need security to find her and remove her. Please. Call me back if you get this message."

He hung his head, dejected. So close yet so far. He ran out of things to do. He went outside and decided to walk down to the quay from where the ship had left hours earlier. He racked his brain for something to do. Anything else he could do.

Legal assistance. He was a lawyer. Who had jurisdiction? The Coast Guard. He checked his phone. Search and rescue was performed by the Australian Volunteer Coast Guard, but crime was managed by the Maritime Border Command, specifically the Royal Australian Navy Patrol Force. He searched the net for a number.

They had a tipline, but if he needed someone to liaise with them, it would be the U.S. embassy. He called them first. The legal office was actually the FBI, but it was the weekend. No one would be working, but he called anyway. There was an emergency phone number in Sydney and one for afterhours.

"State your emergency," the voice answered.

"My girlfriend has been kidnapped and taken to a cruise ship where she's being held against her will. The ship left port without knowing that she was kidnapped and now she's stuck on board." He gave the lady answering the phone the name of the ship.

"Your name?"

"Sterling Bower. I have tickets for us to fly out of Sydney in three days."

"Number where we can contact you and where are you staying?"

He gave her his phone number and the name of the hotel, which was equidistant between the quay and the hospital.

"I'll call if we learn something," the voice promised, but it was a U.S government official, so it sounded hollow. She ended the call.

Sterling felt as helpless as when he found out Stephanie was going on a cruise with Jeremy. He threw all caution to the wind and raced to meet her on the ship in Australia. Good thing, too, but now even that had slipped through his fingers.

He returned to his plan of walking down to the quay and staring longingly at the space where the ship had been berthed.

"HONEY, I'M HOME!" CHIP called joyfully. "I'm cooking dinner."

"Oh really?" Nyla said, coming into the entryway from the living room. She was going to ask what they were having, but Chip carried two takeout bags from an Indian restaurant nearby. The smell reached her. "Ah, curry. My favorite."

"It's both our favorite..." His face fell with the vibration in his pocket. He removed his phone. The hospital. "Doctor McClure."

"Your patient, Stephanie Trent, is on her way in via emergency medevac. She's febrile and jaundiced. She's also in a coma."

Chip closed his eyes and sighed. It would have been so easy to operate this morning. How quickly her fortunes had changed.

"How long until she's at the hospital?"

"Estimate is fifteen minutes from the ship and thirty minutes back to the hospital."

"On my way. Gather my team, if you can. I'll meet them in the O.R."

Nyla had put out two plates but was already returning one to the cupboard.

"Enjoy the curry. The patient from this morning who refused the surgery because she felt better? She's on her way back in and this time, she's dying. I have to go."

"I know you do. I'll stop by the hospital tomorrow to beg them for a job."

"You're highly qualified. You won't have to beg." Chip kissed her and then ran for the door, leaving behind the allure of a good curry. There would be leftovers, but the reheated versions never tasted as good as those right from the restaurant.

The best part of the day had come and gone, but the afternoon showed promise. Too bad Chip would spend it on a road he'd just traveled, going to a place he just left, to do the thing that he should have done earlier this morning.

---

MIRIAM SAW THE NOTE pop up on her app. Stephanie Trent in a coma, inbound via medevac helicopter for emergency surgery at Westpark. Miriam stared at her phone in disbelief. She was fine when she walked out of the hospital this morning.

Her first thought was that Jeremy had done something.

Then reality hit closer to home. When the surgery changed from necessary and covered to elective and not covered, it had made Stephanie's decision much easier.

What if that was the trigger that put her in harm's way and drove costs way up by now including a helicopter ride out to the ship and back? That could cost tens of thousands of dollars. Miriam had upgraded Stephanie's coverage on a whim.

Or was it something else, something like guilt and a gut feeling that the worst was yet to come?

Miriam pushed her coffee cup aside. She closed her list of people to call and left to summon an Uber. It was Sydney. They were never more than ten minutes away, especially on a Sunday with nothing big going on in town. The Ashes was weeks away. A cricket match, one of five to determine the winner between Australia and England, harkening back over a century when Australia won, much to everyone's surprise. Ever since, the competition had been fierce and well attended. It didn't shut down the city, but it occupied a great deal of attention.

Miriam had not been in Sydney during the previous competition, but she'd been warned. She was an American and had no idea what cricket was all about. She only knew that it could take up to five days to play a single match. She barely tolerated the two and a half hours it took to play a game of NFL football.

The Uber kept updating that it was delayed until it finally canceled. She ordered another one. Fifteen minutes. Time was wasting. Stephanie would get to the hospital, and Miriam would be absent. Her guilty conscience was screaming at her.

She called Sterling. "You haven't heard?"

"Heard what? I'm sitting down at the harbor, lamenting my life."

"Stephanie is on her way to Westpark. She's being medevaced off the ship for emergency surgery. I have no further information."

Without hesitation, Sterling replied, "I'll meet you at the hospital. Where would a helicopter deliver a patient?"

"Rooftop landing pad." Miriam had seen one land there before. She hadn't seen one on the grounds outside the hospital.

"I'll meet you in the O.R. waiting room."

"That's where I'm headed." By the time she finished speaking, Sterling had already ended the call.

---

"TIME TO MOVE HER upstairs," the doctor said. Jeremy stayed close to the gurney while the doctor and nurse moved Stephanie onto it and strapped her down. They rolled her over the threshold and into the corridor. The freight elevator was nearby.

The doctor had joked with Stephanie about having two men, saying she was a legend. He was sorry for that. Jeremy was not the man anyone needed to be associated with. And there he was, following closely. Could the doctor get him excluded from the flight and then remain on the ship with him?

Doctor Van Liet had never known the fear that crept up inside him. Jeremy was calm, collected. He seemed perturbed at the one thing he was not in control of, and that was Stephanie's health. How much suffering had she endured before she could take it no longer?

They reached the area near the landing pad, which was forward in a crew-only area on the ship. It was a place where the crew could lounge on deck without interacting with passengers while they were off shift. The sanctity of the passenger areas remained intact. There were no places for employees to grouse about the conditions or the passengers, but they could do that on the landing pad. There were no chairs, but they could bring one of their own or sit on the deck and lean against the forward bulkhead. They could lean on the rail, too.

But with a helicopter inbound, the area had been cleared. They waited with the gurney near steps that led up. The paramedics would carry the gurney the rest of the way and load it onto the helicopter. A telephone connected the area with the bridge. The doctor picked it up. There was no way to dial. It only went to one place.

"Doctor Van Liet with patient, standing by. Advise ETA."

"Five minutes," the bridge replied.

"Copy, five minutes. Out." He spoke like he was military and using a radio, but many of the shipboard operations required navy-like precision. There wasn't room for misunderstandings.

The doctor turned to the nurse.

"Five minutes," she said. "Got it."

The nurse checked Stephanie's pulse and blood pressure. "Pulse one-forty. BP is eighty over forty."

"She's getting worse."

"What could happen next?" Jeremy asked.

"Septicemia. The infection is probably already in her liver, and it'll attack her organs through her bloodstream. The shock will shut her body down."

"You mean she could die?"

"Which is what I've been saying since we found her."

"I found her and reported that she was sick."

It was the first time Jeremy presented anything that appeared to be a legally defensible position. Once again, he stared at the doctor without blinking. If he flew off the ship, the doctor would feel safer.

If Jeremy went to Sydney with Stephanie, then she wouldn't be safe, unless the doctor called ahead and warned them. But what could they do? The doctor had no proof. He only had his feelings and the odd conversations that no one else had heard. He'd sound like he was paranoid, a raving lunatic.

They stood awkwardly waiting, the doctor refusing to look at Jeremy, who refused to look anywhere but the doctor.

The sound of the chopper didn't reach them until it had nearly landed. A crewman ran past with small flags to guide the aircraft in. The ship maintained a slow and steady speed that made the landing pad more accessible. It eased in from a forty-five-degree angle and settled into place following the crewman's direction. Left, right, descend. It came down fairly hard. One of the flight crew, also a paramedic, jumped out and threw a pair of chocks around the tires.

He helped the other paramedic extricate their wheeled stretcher, and they rushed to the stairs.

"We'll move her to ours. It fits in the bird," the first paramedic said. He locked the wheels when the stretchers were side by side. The doctor, nurse, and two paramedics grabbed hold of the sheet beneath Stephanie and slid her across. They strapped her down while Doctor Van Liet secured her paper medical file in a pouch on the side of the stretcher.

"Room for one," the paramedic offered.

"I'll go," Jeremy said. "I'm her husband."

The doctor raised his eyebrows at the claim but said nothing.

"Fine. Time to go. Keep your head down." The paramedics lifted the stretcher up the stairs, rolled it across the landing pad, and slid it into the helicopter, collapsing the wheels and support carriage as it went. They locked it into place and climbed aboard. They pointed to a seat near Stephanie's feet. The paramedics took one next to the pilot and one by Stephanie's head. There were three helmets hooked into the aircraft's comm system so the passengers could talk if needed.

They closed the doors, and the helicopter took off.

"Doctor?" the nurse asked. It was the full question without extra words getting in the way.

"I'll call the surgeon," the doctor said. Even if it made him sound like a nutcase, Chip McClure had seen some of the aberrant behavior firsthand. He wouldn't discount Van Liet's concerns. At least, that's what the doctor hoped.

---

"WE'RE A WAYS OUT to sea so the flight in will take about thirty minutes. Sit back and relax," someone said over the comm system.

Jeremy glanced around the aircraft, at the pilot, at the paramedics, and at Stephanie. He finally looked out the window and watched the ship quickly receding as it steamed toward the open ocean. The water fell far below them.

Despite the minor vibration and the loud engine, greatly muffled by the headset, it was a calm ride. Jeremy wondered if he might take a nap. He'd had a couple drinks while playing cards. The rush of events was taking its toll, although it was nothing he couldn't handle. He'd stay awake as long as it took to see this through.

If Stephanie pulled through, they wouldn't believe anything she said while delusional from the infection and the fever. If she didn't pull through, he'd remember the good times they had.

And then he'd move on.

Once the cruise was finished, of course. It was paid for, and he'd had a great run of luck at the card table. His luck had not yet run out. He was still riding the wave.

And Stephanie? She could join his exaltations and bask in his greatness. Coming along for the ride with him should have been an honor. He needed to remind her of that, if she woke up. He was here for her. She'd see that. He had kept her safe.

Not that other guy. He'd abandoned her in her time of greatest need. He had left the ship and bought plane tickets home.

What a loser! Jeremy smiled at the thought. He'd won, even if Stephanie didn't pull through. He'd still won.

TRAFFIC HAD GOTTEN HEAVY. Chip wasn't sure he was going to make it before the patient arrived. He called the hospital.

"Doctor McClure here, is Nurse Smart there? She is. Good. She'll prep the O.R. for emergency surgery on a patient of mine. Please tell her that we will do the ERCP in the O.R. so that if necessary, we can then proceed to laparotomy. I'm stuck in traffic but on my way. I'll be ready to start as soon as I get there. Please pass the word and thank you." ERCP was an acronym for Endoscopic Retrograde Cholangio Pancreatography.

He wouldn't let them wonder what had happened to him, although if the patient arrived and he wasn't there yet, they'd call. They were never afraid to call, it seemed.

Sometimes at the most inopportune times.

His stomach growled. He had protein bars in his desk for just such an occasion. It wasn't the fine curry he'd left at home, but it calmed the raging innards. He wouldn't have time to eat anything more substantive.

He called the hospital. "Do you have an update on the condition of Miss Trent?"

"Latest was pulse one-forty, blood pressure eighty over forty. They have administered an IV and pushed broad-spectrum antibiotics, specifically ceftriaxone. She's on supplemental O-two."

"That's about all we can do for now. We need to remove that blockage so she can start healing herself. Thank you." Chip hung up. His phone rang immediately.

"Chip, this is Van Liet from the cruise ship. I've sent Stephanie Trent your way, but I have to warn you..." He hesitated.

Chip filled in the rest of the sentence. "She's in bad shape. I just heard the latest."

"She is in bad shape, but that's not what I need to warn you about. That man, Jeremy, is with her. I think he left her to die and then had second thoughts. She was in her room alone, in a coma, for what we think was three hours. The phone had been disconnected so she couldn't call for help before she passed out. I'm concerned about what he might do, but I don't want to sound like a lunatic."

Chip blew out a breath. "That's a serious allegation. That guy gave me the creeps, but I'm not sure I'd call him complicit in her illness or an attempted murderer." He hurried through a light, and the traffic opened up. He was able to start making progress toward the hospital. "He's coming on the chopper with her?"

"He told the paramedics he was her husband."

"He's not, is he?"

"Not as far as I know. I think he wants to be there if she wakes up and starts talking. He'll say she's delusional."

Chip jammed on the brakes. Traffic was back to a full-stop. He hated driving in the city.

"Is she?"

"She was in a coma from the second I found her, after she'd been on board for five hours. He said he was gone for three of those. I think it might have been longer. She would have presented symptoms before he disappeared on her."

The air hung heavy with the weight of what the ship's doctor was saying.

"There's not much I can do about him, but I promise he won't be allowed near the O.R. I'll let security know to keep an eye on him, prevent him from going where he shouldn't. Thanks for the heads up. I'll take it from here, well, as soon as I get to the hospital. I'm stuck in traffic."

"And I'm stuck on a ship getting farther and farther from my patient. For some reason, I care what happens to her." The concern in his voice came through despite the shaky connection from the ship.

"Me, too, my friend. You can count on me to do my best. I'm surrounded by good people. Together, we'll do everything that can be done for her."

The signal blanked out, and the call ended.

Chip stared at the traffic ahead. He felt like parking and running, except he was still too far away.

# CHAPTER EIGHTEEN – INCONGRUITY

STERLING REACHED THE HOSPITAL first. He ran up the stairs instead of waiting for the elevator and then realized he wasn't going to the second floor. He ran back down the stairs and through a corridor, following the signs to the emergency room.

For a moment, he had forgotten where he was. Surgery was one level up from the emergency room, which was on the ground floor. First floor was the first floor above the ground. He pushed through the stairway door and walked back up the steps like a normal human being. His emotions were overwhelming his logical mind. He reached the operating room waiting area, but no one was there, not a nurse behind the desk or a person waiting. It was Sunday, so there wouldn't have been a regularly scheduled operation. There would only be emergencies, and the only emergency had not yet arrived.

He stood at the counter, hoping that someone would see him, but no one arrived.

Sterling called Miriam. "I'm here, but no one else is. Not a surgical team or receiving nurse or anyone."

"I'll be there in five. We'll find out what's going on then. Try to relax and please, don't break anything."

Sterling snorted. "I'm calm, all things considered. Concerned more than anything. Are they bringing her here to Westpark? You're certain?"

"That's what my notification said, but something could have changed. We'll find out when I get there. I know people in the hospital. Try to be patient."

The last thing Sterling wanted was the first thing he had to do. He wanted answers, all of them, and he wanted them yesterday.

---

MIRIAM ENDED THE CALL.

She'd had a feeling that the worst was yet to come, but the issues were spiraling out of control. What if they didn't bring Stephanie to Westpark? What if a different doctor had to perform the surgery? What if she didn't even make it to the table?

She had decided on the light rail because a quick app check showed traffic was clogging the city. Nothing stood in the way of the city's light rail system. She watched as the tram sailed past intersections filled with cars and more behind them, creating a nearly impenetrable morass of humanity in their convenience machines.

The best convenience was a combination of light rail and noise-canceling headphones. With her AirPods blocking out extraneous noise, she continued to pore through Stephanie's records and the policy Miriam had upgraded her to.

The cost of the medevac helicopter was covered under the upgrade but not the previous one.

The emergency surgery and a modicum of recovery time. The upgrade gave Stephanie all the coverage she needed, but policy changes took thirty days before they were in force to prevent someone from doing what Miriam had done. Change a policy for an impending condition without paying the increased premiums that would offset the cost. Pre-existing conditions usually weren't covered.

How could she argue for immediate implementation of the new policy? She'd have time to think about it, but she also had access to a lawyer. He was a criminal lawyer, but shaping arguments was what he did, even though he didn't usually deal with administrative law or medical liabilities. Or maybe he did? How were victims covered when perps committed the crime? Did they have to pay for themselves because perps usually had no money or insurance coverage?

Too many questions and no answers. Her confidence that Stephanie was being brought to Westpark was waning. She knew nothing besides the original report.

Miriam watched for her stop. It was coming up next. She stood and worked her way toward the doors. The day had been a whirlwind of staying busy when there was nothing to do, followed by the race to meet a dying patient that Miriam wouldn't even talk with.

They'd take her straight to surgery.

Why? What was she suffering from? Miriam assumed it was her gallbladder, but assumptions made for poor reporting.

Maybe the doctor would know more. She checked her digital rolodex and there it was, a phone number for Doctor Chip McClure.

She called it.

"McClure," the man answered.

"Chip, this is Miriam Kiryakova. A patient of our mutual interest is headed your way. Stephanie Trent. I'm on my way to the hospital to get in front of this so she gets the care she needs without anyone having to worry."

"That's nice of you," Chip replied. "I'm on my way to the hospital now but am caught in traffic."

"It doesn't get any better closer to the hospital. I'm on the light rail myself. That was the best choice. I'll be to the hospital within a few minutes. Do you know why Stephanie needs emergency surgery?"

Chip sighed. He didn't want to say anything about the patient until he could confirm he was talking with Miriam and not some reporter or investigator trying to trap him into revealing confidential patient information. That would be a crappy thing to do, but he wouldn't put it past a bored journalist.

He was angry at himself for thinking such a thing, but they'd get to the hospital soon enough and could get the information from administration.

"I can't talk about that since I haven't seen the record. Those should be traveling with her. I'll also need to evaluate her myself." That was only partially true. She'd already had about ninety percent of what Chip needed to know. He'd verify for himself, but he was already planning the surgery.

A blocked bile duct. The best method to clear it was by going through the mouth via an endoscope. He wouldn't even have to make an incision. The thing that made the surgery tricky was that she was in such bad shape because of the presumed septicemia. Pump more antibiotics until he could stop the release of toxins from the liver by clearing the duct. Sepsis was imminent the longer they took to operate.

"I'll be waiting at the hospital," Miriam said.

"Wait," Chip interrupted when he felt she was going to end the call. "That man is coming with her. Jeremy. That's his name."

"Oh, God," Miriam said. "If only I could carry pepper spray, I'd probably have reason to use it." She didn't expound. "Thanks for the heads up. Sterling isn't going to like that. I expect fireworks. Is there any place to get popcorn in the hospital?"

"The gift shop," Chip replied honestly but naively.

"I'll stop there first. See you soon." She ended the call. She was getting nowhere with the surgeon regarding Stephanie, but the revelation about the creepy man who had been making eyes at Miriam while his so-called girlfriend was sick made her skin crawl. And he was on his way to the hospital.

---

A CAR SIGNALED TO pull out of a parking spot. Chip waved at him to go. It took a minute for enough space to clear for a single vehicle to get into traffic in front of him. Chip pulled into the spot. He backed up and straightened his car, then turned it off, checked the mirror to make sure no one was coming, and climbed out. He locked the car and started jogging toward the nearest light rail station.

He was too far to run all the way to the hospital. He would if he had to, but that would delay the surgery by another hour.

Chip wasn't the fastest runner, and even pedestrians had to wait for the lights in this part of Sydney. He resigned himself to being late but vowed that he would get there as quickly as possible. He had to take one line for two stops and then switch to another line and take it for two more stops. Then he'd be at the hospital. Ten to fifteen minutes more was all it was going to take once he caught the first tram.

Chip waited for the light. Down the street, he saw a tram pulling into the station. As soon as the light changed, he sprinted across. A late car driven by a frustrated driver pushed to get through the intersection against the yellow and then the red. He slammed on his brakes. Chip dodged to the side, but he was too late.

---

"LANDING IN TWO," THE pilot reported.

Jeremy reached for his harness, but the paramedic stopped him. "Wait until we're on the pad. Landing is where you need to be belted in."

Jeremy knew that. He wanted to get out, stay in front of the situation, whatever that meant. Hanging back in the helicopter wasn't the answer.

The paramedic checked Stephanie's pulse and blood pressure. "Pulse one-fifty. BP is seventy over forty." The paramedic tapped Jeremy's leg. "Stay out of the way. We're going to be running the second we touch down."

Jeremy keyed his microphone. "What's that mean?"

"It means we're lucky she's not dead, mate. Time is not on her side. Now, stay out of the way." The paramedic held eye contact with Jeremy long enough to ensure that he understood.

The man was bigger and appeared to be in better shape. Jeremy had already sized him up as a young man who worked hard for a living. His wasn't a profession for the physically weak.

Not that Jeremy wanted to fight him, only intimidate him into going along with whatever Jeremy wanted to do. Though, he didn't know what that was. Would he be better off if Stephanie died or not?

The question had layers of complexity that Jeremy couldn't completely unravel. If she passed, he'd have to answer questions about leaving her in the room, but ignorance was a viable defense. He wasn't a doctor. He couldn't be held responsible.

If she survived and told what he did to her, taking her passport and locking her in the room, then he'd have more to answer for. A joke? No one would buy that. It was a way to keep her from leaving with Sterling. She still wouldn't leave with him.

Sterling Bower. A quiet man who was a constant reminder that Stephanie had other men. Not just that, but he was in Jeremy's face. Who did that? It was more than annoying. It was aggressive and confrontational. It wasn't something Jeremy could let slide, and he hadn't. Stephanie had gone with him on the ship after a pleasant lunch and a few drinks.

Yes. She had gone with him. She was only feigning a desire to leave the ship. It's because she was sicker than she let on. She left the hospital so she could be with Jeremy.

He relaxed. That story made the most sense to him. If she lived, it would be the one he told her and anyone who would listen. If she didn't, it would still be the story he told. The proof was in her actions.

And on her cell phone. She'd sent Sterling a message. It was as if she'd dictated it to Jeremy and he typed it up for her. Her phone was still in the room. That doctor was going to cause trouble. He was profoundly against Jeremy and Stephanie. He'd called Sterling to her bedside. He tried to deny Jeremy access to the love of his life. He was in the way, but he was also sailing toward Cairns. He'd be out of sight and out of reach for another two days.

This would be resolved by then.

In Jeremy's three-dimensional chess match, the ship's doctor had been taken out of play. He only had to deal with Sterling, maybe that hot insurance agent, and then the surgeon. He had been indifferent to Jeremy's plight. Maybe the E.R. doctor, too.

Enemies. They were all enemies.

A building appeared nearby as the helicopter thumped onto the rooftop landing pad of Westpark Hospital.

# CHAPTER NINETEEN – CONFLUENCE

MIRIAM HURRIED DOWN THE corridor to find Sterling pacing in the waiting room.

"I saw a helicopter landing on the roof," she said without preamble.

He looked up at the ceiling as if he could see to the top floor and beyond. "Which elevator will they use?"

She pointed at the entrance to the surgical ward, the double-doors that were closed and secured. "It's in there. We won't see her."

"Do you know anything? What's wrong with her? What are they going to do and when? There's nobody here."

A nurse hurried past, behind the closed doors. The narrow window showed that it wasn't empty. Sterling raised a fist over his shoulder to pound on the door but paused. The last thing he wanted to do was distract those who would be helping Stephanie. He let his fist drop.

"I might need some legal help," Miriam started.

"Now?" Sterling gestured toward the surgical ward.

"It's about Stephanie's policy. She had coverage for an emergency, but when surgery became elective, it was no longer covered. I don't know why, maybe I had a feeling, but I upgraded her policy to the premier level to cover her for the rest of the trip. I'll drop the coverage back to normal before the bill comes due, but here's where I need help. Policy changes take thirty days to go into effect, but I can guarantee Unified International won't want to pay anything for this."

"That makes no sense to me." Sterling stayed near the window where he could see into a small part of surgery, hoping to catch a glimpse of Stephanie and see that she was being attended to by the sharpest minds and keenest hands.

"If she had had the emergency surgery, then everything would have been fine, but she claimed she felt better, which made it elective and that wasn't covered. You see where I'm going with this?"

Sterling nodded. "They'll make their case based on patient's refusal to do what was best, which increased the cost of the procedure astronomically coupled with the upgrade in coverage, which has a so-called cooling off period to keep people from knowing they have some debilitating disease and changing their coverage before their condition is known, and their rates skyrocket because of it. The pool of money still has a fair-share cost basis. No one gets coverage that has a million-dollar impending procedure for the same price as those who are perfectly healthy. Shareholder value depends on more of the latter and fewer of the former."

"You've encapsulated the entirety of the insurance industry in a few sentences. I want this to be paid for, so Stephanie doesn't have a bill waiting for her when she recovers, a bill she can't pay."

"So, she is going to be okay?" Sterling stared at Miriam, who threw up her hands.

"I don't know. I always presume the patient will be saved. Stephanie is young and strong, I feel that in my soul, and she's on her way for the best people to see her."

Sterling returned to staring at the window and into a single corridor that ended at a T-intersection.

Somewhere in there, they were preparing to operate on Stephanie.

"I need to think." Sterling was lost in unknowns. He didn't know the policy. He didn't know the applicable laws. He couldn't reference any cases. And most importantly, he had no idea how Stephanie was. "I have to see her, hold her hand. She'll know I'm there."

"You're not going to get in there." Miriam stepped in front of him. "You have to let them do their job."

---

THE PARAMEDIC IN THE co-pilot's seat jumped out first and placed the chocks on one of the bird's wheels. The other paramedic opened the side door. He released the locking clamps that held the stretcher in place. A doctor and a nurse waited in a building to the side of the pad. It was enclosed, and that's where the elevator was to take patients from the rooftop delivery to whoever needed to see them. In this case, it was the ground floor and the emergency room, despite the urgency for surgery.

The E.R. team would make sure the patient needed surgery. They would do their best to stabilize her and then send her upstairs once the need was confirmed. It didn't have to take long. That was time the surgical team needed to prep. Some things could be hurried, while other things took time out of necessity. Performing an unnecessary surgery because of suppositions didn't help anyone. Guessing was the last thing a patient needed. Educated guesses? Those happened all the time, but they were made with as much information as possible.

They rushed the stretcher across the landing pad and to the waiting elevator. The paramedics let the doctor and nurse take the patient, and they waited behind.

"We'll follow," the first paramedic promised. They had paperwork to complete, but the patient was always the priority.

Jeremy squeezed in with them. It wasn't that small of a space. The paramedics probably could have fit, but if they needed to perform CPR or more immediate procedures on the patient, there wouldn't have been room.

The doctor and nurse checked for obs. Before they reached the emergency room, they confirmed the broad-spectrum antibiotics.

"Add one gram of piperacillin and tazobactam," the doctor ordered. "Get me surgery."

"Right away, Doctor," a receiving nurse said. The doctor and nurse pushed the stretcher into a room where a nurse and a lab tech waited.

"Standard battery of blood tests as part of surgical prep. She's about to experience septic shock. We need to get that bile duct cleared and the gallbladder addressed. Need an ultrasound to verify the stone migrated." Stephanie's blood pressure appeared on a monitor above the bed. "Hurry up, people. We're losing her."

Jeremy stood just inside the opening to the room, staying out of the way. When the doctor took a one-second breather, he noticed him.

"You'll have to wait outside. Nurse!" The doctor gestured for Jeremy to leave. He wandered into the hallway but then stood there watching the doorway. He'd already seen this play out yesterday, but they let him stay, along with too many other people.

"Sir?" A nurse intercepted him. "The waiting room is this way." She blocked him with one arm and pointed the way with the other.

"She needs surgery," Jeremy said woodenly.

"Then they'll take her upstairs. We'll let you know, but you can't be in here. Let the staff do their jobs." She didn't expound with false hope. Even she knew how bad it was. Good thing the E.R. wasn't busy, because nearly everyone was involved with this one patient.

She stood like that, blocking Jeremy from going back in the room while he refused to leave, not in words but with his actions. He remained rooted to the floor.

"I know what you're feeling, we see that too much in here, but you really have to wait outside. I need to be doing things that don't involve you. So, please..." She stabbed a finger at the door.

Jeremy continued to stay where he was.

"Security!" the nurse shouted. She didn't have time to play games or babysit an emotionally shattered loved one.

"Fine," Jeremy conceded. Twice in less than twenty-four hours, he'd been forced to leave the E.R. by means of a security officer. He walked away as the man in uniform appeared and then waited until the doors closed behind him.

Jeremy stood outside the doors, looking inside where he was no longer allowed. When he turned around, he found a young couple with a sniffling child, a man holding his arm, and a distraught woman crying. He moved as far away from all of them as he could get. He had no intention of catching whatever the kid had or joining those in pain or grieving.

It was going to be a while before any of them went into the back. He didn't feel anything for any of them. He had his issues which didn't involve any of them, and they had theirs which didn't involve him.

---

CHIP FOUND HIMSELF ON his back in the middle of the street. Two teenagers leaned over him. One had his hand in Chip's pocket.

"Hey! Get out of there." Chip caught the young man's wrist and squeezed tightly.

"Just looking for identification so we know who to call, but since you're not dead, we'll leave you to it." The two popped up and ran off.

Chip rolled over and struggled to get on his hands and knees. So far so good. He didn't think anything was broken. He managed to get to his feet, which made his hip complain, sending stabbing pains into his leg. He felt his leg. It didn't seem broken, only bruised. He felt his pockets. His wallet was still in place, but his car keys were gone. His golf clubs were still in the trunk. A house key was part of the set. His home address was on the registration in the glovebox. He needed to contact the police. Secure his vehicle. Keep the miscreants from finding it, even though it was two blocks away.

People honked while he stood there. An older woman approached. "Are you okay?" she asked.

"I seem to be mostly okay. Where's the car that hit me?"

She pointed down the road. "It's that red one."

Chip reached for his phone to take a picture of the license plate, but his phone was gone, too. "Can you get a picture of that for me? Seems like the first responders have cleaned me out. At least I have my wallet." He pulled out a business card that he always carried in case he needed someone to follow up with him and he wasn't at his desk.

The older woman complied while cars continued to honk. Chip waved at the drivers while the two of them moved to the sidewalk. He didn't want any more trouble.

"I need to get to the hospital," he said.

"Are you hurt? Do I need to call an ambulance?" the lady offered.

"No. Well, yes, but no. I'm a surgeon and have been called for an emergency. That's why I was rushing. Someone's life is in jeopardy."

"Then you better go." The lady looked at Chip's business card while he thanked her on his way to the light rail station just past the next corner.

He tried to run, but his hip protested. He managed a limping jog, with each step more painful than the last. The tram was long gone, so he didn't need to hurry. He settled for a measured walk, taking shorter steps to minimize the pain. He was already late, and now the hospital couldn't reach him.

Chip was doing the best he could, but that was never an excuse when one's best wasn't good enough. If Stephanie died, he'd blame himself. He rarely lost patients, but he remembered all the names of those who had passed away under his care.

Roo had been a success when it could have easily gone the other way. Now Stephanie. Two patients in a row who needed lifesaving surgery.

Routine. The word that Bethany threw around as if bending it to her will. Very little of Chip's life was routine besides the long hours. His surgeries were laparoscopic or endoscopic. He wasn't up to his elbows in blood. He silently thanked his chosen field for the cleaner elements of his operations. Most, anyway.

Chip limped up to the station. Leaving the scene of an accident would weaken his claim. Inability to call the police would be another strike against him, but if the punks found his car and took it, that would be on them. He'd have to get it rekeyed if they didn't steal it. His house? They wouldn't know where he lived, which made the house key useless unless they found the car, then they'd have his address on the registration. Maybe he'd rekey the house anyway. What a debacle.

He took a seat on the bench. His hip ached even while sitting.

Could he perform the surgery while injured? He'd get an x-ray. It might show a stress fracture of the hip or femoral neck. Either case would require a long rehabilitation period. In other words, it would hurt for a long time to come.

He hung his head.

A homeless person shuffled by, holding out a hat with a few coins inside. Chip didn't have any small bills on him. He held up his hands. Giving money to the homeless was a double-edged sword. They needed help, but was it the help a five- or ten-dollar note could solve? The money might buy alcohol instead of food. How much would it enable them before they decided to turn their lives around? Rock bottom. That's usually what it took before they were forced to change.

It was never easy, not for them and not for society, but without their willingness, no one could force them to cooperate with those who wanted to help. From the hospital to shelters to counselors.

The man moved on after checking over Chip, who was filthy from his roll in the street. His trouser knees were black with street dirt. His arms, too. Even the homeless had given him a pass.

The next tram was coming.

Chip stood, taking his time to get through the pain that threatened to overwhelm him.

*You have to be tougher than this. Stephanie needs you.*

It was the same story he told himself nearly every day. Someone needed him. Nyla was the most accommodating. The look on her face when his phone rang was the same every time. Disappointment. His job provided for their lifestyle, but it was far more than a job. His profession demanded that he adhere to the highest standards of a servant position.

He was always on call. Well, not right now because his phone had been stolen. He snorted at the nature of his life. He was winning, but it didn't feel like it. He needed to get to the hospital. At least he was much closer, despite everything. No calls without a phone. No damage control for his car or his home. No heads up that he'd need to be evaluated and treated.

Once the surgery was done. Without a phone, he would have no information until he was physically in the hospital. If they waited for him. How long would it take to bring in another surgeon who could perform the operation?

Too long, if the last word on Stephanie's vitals was anything to go by.

# CHAPTER TWENTY – PYRE

"CALL HIM AGAIN!" POSSUM Joe said out of frustration. Bethany had already tried three times, and there was no answer.

"I'm calling Nyla," Bethany replied. She dialed the phone, and Nyla answered on the second ring. "Nyla, Bethany here. Do you know where Chip is?"

"On his way to the hospital. He's not there yet?" Nyla replied.

"No. No one's heard from him, and he's not answering his phone."

Nyla paused. "I have a tracking app for his phone. Let me pull up where he is."

Bethany waited.

"He's headed toward Circular Quay? It looks like he's either running or riding a bike since the signal is moving quickly. I don't understand. He was on his way to the hospital."

"All we can do is keep trying to contact him. The only thing we know for sure is that he's not here and the patient is."

Nyla groaned. She hated it when Chip was called in on the weekends, but she also knew how important his job was. The patients needed him, and she tried to be better about sharing her husband with those in need.

"I'll call him."

The phone went dead. "What would he be doing at Circular Quay?" Bethany asked. "He was driving himself, not taking the ferry. I better call for a replacement."

Joe had no idea what was going on. Surgery or no? That was Chip's call and he wasn't here, but everyone else was. They'd started the prep but hadn't scrubbed yet. That would be soon, if the surgery was to happen. Stephanie was in the emergency room getting prepped. If a replacement surgeon was found, it would take forever to get them here. He wondered if the medevac helicopter was still on the roof.

"I'm going downstairs," Joe said. He headed for the stairs while Bethany waited for Nyla to call back. That call came after less than a minute.

"He's not answering. It shows he's on a ferry. I don't know which one."

"You're sure he drove?" Bethany asked.

"I'm sure. His car isn't out there. It's Sunday. He always drives himself on the weekends, unless something is going on in the city. I called twice, quickly, and that's our secret signal that he needs to answer, no matter what's going on. I'm worried, Beth. What can we do?"

"Wait. It's all we can do until he either picks up the phone or someone sees him." Beth ended the call. She knew that Nyla would keep calling and so would Bethany.

She called the main desk. "We need a surgeon who can treat a patient with cholangitis. Our surgeon has gone missing. Please access the on-call list of surgeons and then the other hospitals and see if they have anyone available. The sooner the better."

---

JOE WENT DOWN THE stairs that delivered him directly into the E.R. He had to use his badge to open the door because it was a restricted area. He found them busy, but with only Stephanie. The lab was expediting the blood results, looking for organ function among many other things.

The doctor hovered outside Stephanie's door with a crash trolley ready to bring her back to life if her heart stopped.

"Blood pressure is too low and pulse is too high," the doctor said after greeting Joe.

"We're prepped upstairs, except for one minor thing," Joe said.

"Anything we can provide?"

"Chip McClure? Is he hiding down here somewhere?"

"I haven't seen him. I'm sure you tried calling him."

"No answer, repeatedly. Something has happened to him, and we don't know what."

"Anyone else around who can perform the surgery?"

"Yes, but he's not in Sydney this weekend. They're calling other hospitals right now," Joe explained.

The E.R. doctor stopped a nurse in the hallway. "Please make a public address announcement for Doctor Chip McClure to report to the E.R."

Within a minute, the announcement echoed throughout the hospital.

Joe didn't hold out hope that Chip was in the hospital. "Can I see her?" he asked.

The doctor escorted him in. She had already been intubated in addition to the IV and a heavy dose of antibiotics. Joe looked at her chart first because she looked bad. He checked her eyes, almost like he was obligated. Jaundice. She was hot to the touch, her body attempting to fight the infection that raged through her body.

"Stay with us, Stephanie. A little while longer," he pleaded. He faced the E.R. doctor. "I'll be upstairs, acting like we're going to do this surgery any minute now. We'll be ready for her."

---

JEREMY SAT CALMLY IN the E.R. waiting room but only for so long. Stephanie was in there, and no one was telling him anything. He wanted to know. He *needed* to know. He approached the desk. "Can you give me an update on Stephanie Trent, please?"

"I don't have any new information. I'm sorry." She looked past him. "William Grimes?"

The parents with the toddler approached the desk. The boy coughed with his mouth wide open, not bothering to cover it.

Jeremy dodged out of the way. "Jeez!"

"Sorry," the mother mumbled while the father carried the child, cradling him against his chest.

"You could find out," Jeremy persisted.

"Or they could tell me when there's an update." She gestured for him to go away. There was a note in Stephanie's record that stated he wasn't a relation and was not to be given her medical information.

She glanced at him watching her while she checked in the boy and escorted him into the back.

---

CHIP HEARD THE LAST of the announcement summoning him to the E.R. That was the best place for him, so that's where he went. His limp had grown quite pronounced by the time he reached the check-in desk. He leaned heavily on it, waiting for the nurse to return. His badge would have opened the door to the surgery suite, but he had strained to get to and through the hospital's front doors and needed a short rest.

The nurse returned. "Chip! They've been looking for you..." She stopped when she saw the state of him. "Are you okay?"

"Can you get me a wheelchair?" He surrendered. Trying to walk anymore would only cause him more pain and anguish. He fully intended to perform the surgery.

"Doctor McClure," a familiar voice called from behind him.

Chip pivoted without putting any weight on his bad side to find one of his patient's boyfriends standing there. Jeremy, the one none of them liked.

"How is she? They won't tell me what's going on. You look like hell," Jeremy observed.

The nurse returned with a wheelchair. Chip sat down gingerly.

"I just got here myself. I need to find out what's going on first. Be patient," Chip called over his shoulder as the nurse rolled him through the doors and toward Stephanie's room. She hesitated once through to make sure the doors closed behind her.

Jeremy had tried to follow. He was one step back. Once the door closed, she continued. "Chip is here," she shouted.

The E.R. doctor met him. "What happened to you?"

"No time. How's my patient?"

"Ready to die," the doctor replied without hesitation. "Ultrasound confirms a dilated bile duct, possibly from a stone blocking it. She has cholangitis and is in septic shock. Need to remove that stone, posthaste."

The doctor held out the image from the ultrasound. He showed the lab results. "Is my team here?"

"Just talked with Possum Joe. They're upstairs and prepping as if they knew you were going to make it. They couldn't get a hold of you." The doctor looked into the room. "Time for surgery. Bring her upstairs, please."

Chip nodded. "Phone was stolen—car keys, too—and I was hit by a car. I'll probably be back down here after we take care of Miss Trent. I'll meet her upstairs."

"I'll take him," the doctor said, pushing the wheelchair toward the elevator when Chip tried to roll it himself.

They headed upstairs, and the nurse returned to the front desk.

Chip went straight to the locker room, where he had to get out of the wheelchair and drop his dirty clothes on the floor. He kicked them toward his locker, grimacing from the surge of pain from what should have been simple. He pulled fresh scrubs from the rack. He dressed far more slowly than he usually did, especially considering his patient's circumstances.

Both Joe and Bethany joined him in the locker room. "Since you're here and your phone is on its way across the bay, I'm assuming it was stolen?"

"Along with my car keys, but I caught them before they got my wallet, but none of that matters. Are we ready to remove that stone? An ERCP and sphincterotomy should alleviate matters." Chip was one of the few surgeons in Sydney who had endoscopic as well as laparoscopic and open surgery expertise. This endoscopic procedure allowed for access to the bile duct via an endoscope called a duodenoscope.

"We're set up for the ERCP. You say what you're going to do, and I'll hand you the right tools," Bethany confirmed.

"You're the best, Beth." He took one careful step, grunted, and stopped. "Can I get a hand?"

"Right up until you scrub, then you're on your own. Are you going to make it?"

"That's not a question for me. That's best asked of our patient." He motioned toward the door. "Let's do this."

Chip was confident. He knew what he had to do. He only needed to get into the O.R. and take a seat. He'd do everything he needed from there. He stepped gingerly, doing his best not to limp on his way to scrub up with Beth and Joe.

THE E.R. ADMISSIONS NURSE returned without Chip and without the wheelchair.

Jeremy intercepted her before she could sit down. "Is Steph headed for surgery now that the surgeon is here?"

"I can't tell you. The doctor will make his determination based on the information that's been gathered," she replied noncommittally.

"He is. You could just tell me."

The woman made a face and shrugged. She had no intention of telling him anything.

Jeremy hurried down the hall to the stairs and disappeared inside. He took them two at a time up one floor. A sign on the wall pointed to his right if he wanted to go to the operating room waiting area.

He did. He walked briskly down the corridor, pulling up short when he saw the only two people in there.

"Miriam," he stated coldly before shifting his gaze to Sterling. "You."

"We're not going to fight," Sterling said. "This is all about Stephanie."

"If we did, you'd be on the short end. You are such a loser, Bower. Loser with a capital L."

Miriam looked disgusted. "Did you stop maturing when you turned twelve? Does your entire purpose revolve around going to the beach and kicking sand in people's faces?"

"Women like you need protectors like me. You don't have to say anything. You know it's true. This clown! Desk jockey. He should be charged a tax for how much oxygen he wastes." Jeremy scoffed at Sterling.

"I'm busy," he said and returned to scrolling on his phone. He was using his Lexis/Nexis access to search for applicable case law. There wasn't as much as he hoped, but there were cases regarding patients suing their insurance company for non-payment. What he needed, however, was any case law that revolved around changing diagnoses that went from required to elective and then back to required. The determination of coverage shouldn't be made based on an interim change that then reverted, but he wanted a solid foundation on which to base his premise.

"Playing Words with Friends? Odd, since you don't have any friends," Jeremy tried as the lamest of taunts.

"You have to be the most annoying man I've ever met," Miriam stated.

"That's because you haven't gotten to know me. You'll change your mind. Remember, good protector. Good provider. I'm the whole package, baby."

"You are a festering package of petri dish waste."

Sterling nudged her. "Don't descend to his level. I doubt it's very pretty down there." He lifted his head. "What are you doing here?"

"I came with Stephanie from the ship. The doctor is here, and I think they're starting surgery, but they wouldn't tell me anything. I'm sure they came this way. That surgeon looks like he was run over. They had to move him with a wheelchair."

"They what? He was fine when we saw him yesterday," Miriam said.

"He's not fine now." Jeremy took a seat, one row away from Miriam and Sterling but facing them so he could continue to stare.

Miriam moved to the next row and put her back to him and Sterling. She had no patience for grade school verbal jousting. She needed to find supporting evidence that what she did for Stephanie was okay. Sterling was looking for something that would resonate before a judge, which he could use as precedent for a convincing argument to force the insurance company to pay.

It made sense that they needed to pay because it was an emergency, which meant that it should be paid as a matter of course. Precedent would go a long way in convincing a judge for a summary ruling, should the case advance to that stage. Or Unified International could settle out of court by simply paying the bill.

Worst case and best case. A jury trial was fraught with risk and would be subject to endless delays. A trial before a judge would depend on the forum. A victim-friendly judge would be more easily swayed than a big-business judge. Finding a venue with a more amenable judge was called forum shopping. It wasn't beneath Sterling to do such a thing. Some jurisdictions were hostile to his clients. At least with a neutral location, the case would be tried solely on its merits.

"You haven't checked in on Stephanie, despite your bluster," Jeremy said into the silence.

Sterling wanted to beat Jeremy into next week but was convinced he couldn't take him in a straight-up fight. The man was in much better shape. Jeremy was a bully, and the best way to handle a bully was to confront him, straight on, except that was the grade school approach. As adults, minimizing their influence and crushing their ego delivered the desired result. Get them to go away.

"Don't you have a puppy you need to kick?" Sterling said without looking up. He had no sway in the hospital, but Miriam had said she knew people. He was waiting for her to pull strings and get the latest on Stephanie.

He had work to do, which kept his mind busy and would serve Stephanie in the end. If he thought about what she was going through, it would wear him down. He'd crumble into an incoherent puddle. That would help no one. At least he could think he was making a difference by researching and taking notes. He would have preferred his computer, but that was in the hotel. He had come straight to the hospital without stopping to get anything.

It was okay. Once she was in recovery, he'd give more than one hundred percent of his focus to Miriam's concerns. If Sterling couldn't build a compelling case, he'd find someone who could. He had a lot of peers from law school and a network of professionals to ask for help. He'd get a great response if he was willing to pay.

Busy people were the best at getting things done, especially when there were dollar signs attached.

*My kingdom for a horse*, Sterling thought.

The low-battery indicator flashed. He'd been ignoring it, but his phone was down to five percent.

"Do you have a phone charger?" he whispered over his shoulder at Miriam.

"Oddly enough, I do. And to think that men make fun of purses, but when you need something, who do you go to?"

"I don't make fun of purses. I carry a briefcase in my day job. Same thing, but it has the benefit of a manly name."

Miriam chuckled. She handed over a plug with a short USB-C cable. Sterling found an outlet on the wall and moved seats so he could plug in and continue to research.

Jeremy glared at them. He also moved seats, so he could see Miriam's face.

"What is wrong with you?"

"You don't have a man, do you?" he asked.

She didn't—not at the moment—but that was irrelevant. 'Having a man,' as Jeremy put it, was her choice and not in any way a compliment under Jeremy's sordid definition of roles and responsibilities. She didn't need a protector, as he had called himself. She'd be glad of a partner she could laugh and share life's adventure with.

Wasn't that what most people wanted out of a relationship?

"That doesn't justify a response. Has anyone told you what a pig you are?"

"So, no, then." He smirked while staring at her.

It was time to find out what was going on, and that meant getting away from Jeremy.

She leaned close to Sterling. "You're on your own," she told him and walked out.

# CHAPTER TWENTY-ONE – DETAILS

Miriam went straight to the emergency room, where she stood at the check-in desk and waited for the admissions nurse to return. Miriam knew her and more importantly, the nurse knew Miriam.

She showed her insurance agent identity card, which granted her access to her client's records. Just to stay above board in case Jeremy showed up and demanded the same information. But he hadn't followed her. She had taken the long way, stopping by the bathroom to throw him off.

"She's been moved upstairs to surgery, but I have to warn you not to get your hopes up. That's just between us girls. The doctors will do all they can. It would have been better if she had been brought in hours earlier."

Miriam hung her head. "There will be questions about why it took so long, but for now, it just did, and Stephanie is the one to suffer the consequences of the delay. I'll pray that Chip and his team can deliver a miracle."

---

CHIP, BETHANY, AND JOE scrubbed up and pulled their gloves tight. Unlike other forms of surgery, endoscopic surgery did not require wearing masks.

Abby held Stephanie's limp hand while Joe monitored her response to the medication. Sedating an unconscious patient carried risks. How much was too much, and how much was too little?

It was the professional's job to determine the correct dose.

Chip moved slowly into his chair. It would not be easy doing the procedure sitting, however, he was very experienced. Many of his colleagues had commented that he would be able to carry out endoscopic surgery even if he was upside-down.

They turned Stephanie onto her left side. Chip introduced the duodenoscope through the mouth guard that had been placed to keep her mouth open and navigated the 'scope into the duodenum so that the opening of the bile duct, the papilla, was visible. Obvious pus was exuding from the opening, which confirmed the severity of her condition.

As he was about to introduce instruments to help visualize the bile duct and the cause of the obstruction, he heard Joe shout, "I'm losing her. The heart has stopped! Chip, you have to stop!"

---

STERLING HAD DONE AS much as his eyes could handle using his phone. Lexis/Nexis wasn't the easiest database to use, and the small screen only exacerbated the difficulties.

U.S. case law referenced medical necessity—a definition provided by an independent group of advisors for each condition. If the patient met all the conditions, then the procedure was medically necessary. It wasn't an objective standard.

*The patient will suffer from, or has a high chance of suffering from, a significant deterioration in health-related wellbeing, or continuation of a significantly lower than normal state of health-related wellbeing.*

But for the procedure, the patient's condition would worsen considerably with negative long-term health impacts or death.

He considered death a negative long-term impact, although he would have appreciated that it was listed separately. Procedures to save a life were usually medically necessary. The drawback was that too many doctors ordered procedures that weren't completely necessary. Most doctors had zero incentive to control costs. In fact, they were incentivized to minimize risk for their patients because of malpractice lawsuits, which sometimes held doctors to a god-like standard for diagnosis and prognosis. The doctor was allowed little latitude to get it wrong from a reasonable-person standard.

The insurance industry was big business, and when the almighty dollar and a nobody patient collided, the patient tended to lose.

Sterling watched Miriam's crusade to ensure Stephanie was taken care of. Unified International Healthcare had deep pockets. They could have afforded the earlier procedure, which would have saved them a great deal of money rather than the later emergency procedure and threat of death. If she died, that was a life insurance problem and not a healthcare problem. It was horrible to think that the insurance company would prefer patients died to the long-term costs of recovery when it came to more severe issues.

If Stephanie survived, how long would her recovery take?

*If...* The thought caught in Sterling's throat. He'd always assumed she would be there. He hadn't taken her for granted—at least, he didn't think he had—but she had moved on without him. That's how Jeremy came into her life.

*Let's do something fun that's not staying at home,* he thought, committing to asking her *when* she recovered. Driving the Iowa countryside. Taking back roads. Getting lost. And loving every minute of it. His eyes glazed as he contemplated everything he was about to lose.

Costs were the least of his problems. He tried to go back to researching, but he couldn't see. The world was blurry. He wiped his eyes on his sleeves.

"Pansy," Jeremy said from nearby.

Sterling had forgotten where he was. The waiting room. Stephanie was on the other side of those doors with a surgeon racing to save her. All his skill and experience to perform the procedure in the least amount of time in the best way, avoid things that caused more harm while doing everything else. Sterling was just a lawyer. He worked with words and research. The surgeon worked with his hands, eyes, and intelligence. He adjusted on the fly.

Sterling rarely had to deal with changes where he had to react. If he did his job properly, there were no surprises. Don't ask a question you don't already know the answer to. It was an easy premise to understand but hard in reality. Every case required a meticulous breakdown of all possible moves and then memorization of the countermoves, including the applicable case law.

Insurance company non-payment didn't have much case law supporting it. The insurance companies had batteries of lawyers, while the aggrieved had nothing but mounting medical debt. They couldn't afford to sue.

And that added to the shareholders' bottom line.

Sterling's lip curled at the thought. He unplugged the charger and rolled up the cable to stuff it in his pocket. He carried his phone in his hand. "I need some air," he told Jeremy, even though he owed the man nothing.

He owed him less than nothing. He didn't know why he said anything.

Sterling was letting the bully win.

"When you get outside, why don't you keep walking. She won't want to see you since you abandoned her. Yesterday, today, and might as well throw in tomorrow, too."

"You live in an interesting world, Jeremy. A fantasy world where you rule over everything you see. I pity you." Sterling strode toward the stairs while Jeremy talked, saying nothing of import, spewing more nonsense.

Sterling was better off outside, but he wouldn't go far. Miriam was somewhere. He knew she wouldn't leave while Stephanie was in surgery. He guessed she was finding out what was going on, getting an update while Sterling was barely keeping it together.

His issues were nothing compared to what Stephanie was going through. He made it outside and found a bench in the sun. He wasn't a religious man, but he closed his eyes and prayed.

# CHAPTER TWENTY-TWO – FURTHERANCE

MIRIAM RETURNED TO THE surgery waiting room but turned around when she saw Jeremy and hurried away. Where had Sterling gone? She wanted to update him with what she had learned, even though it wasn't much.

Maybe it was enough to give him hope. The simple fact that Stephanie was still alive had to be enough, because it was all she had.

She went downstairs, intending to go to the cafeteria, but she saw Sterling with his shoulders slumped and his head bowed on a bench near the main entrance to the private side of the massive hospital.

The weather was congenial and warm, a break from the cool of recent rainstorms. The sun beat down on him, but he ignored it, not opting to move into the shade.

"Sterling," Miriam interrupted the man's thoughts. "She's still with us. Chip is operating on her. She's young and a fighter." Miriam didn't know why she added that last part, probably to reassure herself more than Sterling. She sat on the bench next to him, wincing when the bare skin of her leg touched the hot surface. "That's gonna leave a mark," she blurted.

She adjusted her shorts to cover the seat.

"Are you okay?" she asked.

He sat up straight, squinting against the sun. He made a visor with his hand to block the rays. "Not in any way, shape, or form. I've never felt so helpless." He bent over and held his face with his hands.

"There's nothing anyone can do. We'll be there when she wakes up."

"*If...*" Sterling clarified.

"If, but we have to hold out hope. Without hope, what's it all mean?"

He shrugged. The depths of depression summoned him, tearing at his very soul.

"A meeting of the minds?" Jeremy had walked up behind them. "Doesn't this look precious. If I had a phone on me, I would have taken a picture. I'll just have to describe it to Stephanie when she wakes up."

"She's out of surgery?" Miriam wondered. They both stood and faced Jeremy on the other side of the bench.

"How would I know? They aren't telling me anything. I wonder why that is?"

Miriam and Sterling both glared at the man.

Sterling snapped. He growled until it turned into a roar. He stepped on the bench to throw himself over it and onto Jeremy.

Miriam hit him from the side, tackling him. They both bounced off the bench and rolled to the ground.

Sterling's moment of fury had already passed. He knew Miriam had been right in stopping him. "Thanks," he mumbled.

Jeremy roared with laughter. "Look at you two morons. I wish I had a camera for this."

Sterling was first to his feet. He pulled Miriam upright. "Shall we wait inside? It's gotten a bit warm out here." He gave Jeremy a wide berth as he walked with a measured step toward the entrance.

Jeremy stared after Sterling.

Miriam took one step, then swung around, kicking straight up between Jeremy's legs. Her toe thudded upon impact. He gasped and dropped to his knees. She straightened her hair as she walked away, giving her hips an extra swing on her way to the front door.

As a violent criminal, her work visa could be revoked, but anyone who met Jeremy would believe that she was only defending herself. She wouldn't bother mentioning it if he didn't make an issue of it, which he wouldn't because it wouldn't reflect well on his manliness.

"What happened?" Sterling asked from inside the front door.

Jeremy was still on his knees, coughing.

"Football," Miriam replied simply. "He wasn't up for it."

They returned to the emergency room admissions nurse. No patients were in the waiting area. It was empty.

"Anything new?"

"No, honey, but seeing as I'm out of customers at the moment, I'll run upstairs and take a look. You wait right here."

Miriam and Sterling stood there like anxious friends. There was nothing to say, nothing to do. All they could do was fight to be patient and pray that the surgeon would deliver a masterful performance. And that Stephanie had enough fight left in her to pull through. Hope. Miriam had it right. Hopelessness was no way to live.

Time stretched to infinity for every second the nurse was away. No new patients appeared. There was no one new to take advantage of E.R. services. That meant there were no distractions. They couldn't see Jeremy from where they were. Miriam went to the window to look for him. She didn't trust that he wouldn't seek retribution of some sort for the blow she'd delivered to him and his ego.

---

QUICKER THAN WHEN HE inserted the endoscope, Chip deftly removed it so that Stephanie could be turned on her back. Chip pushed himself out of the way so that Joe and the nurses had full access.

Abby started chest compressions, CPR to keep the blood flowing.

The crash trolley was quickly brought into place and the cardiac paddles produced. The endotracheal tube that Joe had previously inserted kept her ventilated, but she needed her heart restarted. Without a heartbeat, oxygen was almost useless.

The cardiac monitor demonstrated a flat line. Abby maintained her rhythm.

"Heartbeat," Joe stated, watching the monitor.

Joe placed the paddles on her chest, exactly as he trained for, ensured that no one was in contact with Stephanie, and activated the device to deliver the charge to regulate her erratic heartbeat. The cardiac monitor showed an instant response as her heart settled into a regular rhythm. Their promptness ensured rapid resuscitation, but Joe knew full well that unless the pus was released from the obstructed bile duct, Stephanie's life was on a knife's edge.

Her heart stopped for a reason. Chip needed to get back in there and remove the cause.

Stephanie was repositioned in the left lateral position, and Chip expertly reinserted the duodenoscope.

"Catheter or sphincterotome?" Bethany asked.

"Sphincterotome, please," Chip replied. He introduced the sphincterotome into the 'scope and as it appeared through the tip of the 'scope, Chip manipulated it into the bile duct. In these instances where there was infection and exuding pus, navigation into the bile duct from the duodenum was relatively straightforward.

The position of the sphincterotome was checked by the infusion of contrast material so that a radiologic image of the duct could be seen on the x-ray monitor.

"Ah! There it is, the offending stone!" Chip exclaimed without being overly excited. He had managed to dislodge the stone from where it had impacted to obstruct the bile duct. Bethany opened the handle of the sphincterotome so that the diathermy wire positioned across the opening of the bile duct became taut. Chip applied bursts of coagulating and cutting current using a foot pedal.

The lower end of the duct, the sphincter of Oddi, was divided, and a flood of pus and bile flowed into the duodenum. Replacing the sphincterotome by a balloon catheter, Chip cleared the duct of stones and pus until there was a free flow of irrigating fluid.

---

SHE DECIDED TO STAY close to Sterling. The two of them together could manage Jeremy and his bullying.

The nurse walked down the corridor toward them. She opened the door and walked through, moving behind her desk before she spoke. "She's still in surgery, and she's still alive. Anything else I could tell you would be conjecture, and I don't want to do that. You're just going to have to wait."

"We'll go upstairs and wait there."

"Why don't you get yourselves something to eat and maybe a cup of coffee. Relax as much as you can and let the doctor work."

"Good advice. Thank you for everything," Miriam told her acquaintance. She ushered Sterling toward the cafeteria, moving slowly and scanning the area.

She was afraid of what Jeremy might do.

Sterling was afraid of what Jeremy had done to Stephanie.

Everyone had an issue with Jeremy.

Sterling chuckled.

Miriam looked at him oddly.

"That freaking guy. What did you do to him? Be honest."

"No." Miriam said no more. The cafeteria had few people, mostly employees in scrubs or other hospital attire. They went to the counter, but nothing looked appealing. Coffee was the order of the day. Dripped out of an oversized urn, much to the disdain of the staff and the ridicule of anyone who saw it.

But they all drank it because it served as a magic elixir and was so bad that friends and enemies alike could rally against it. Unite against the common foe and share tales of drinking it for therapeutic value only. None would admit liking it.

Miriam and Sterling both took a cup. At the register, Miriam selected a single oversized cookie—biscuits, they were called down under.

Sterling stared at it.

"What? I eat cookies when I'm stressed."

Sterling paid for it all. He tried to pay in cash, but it was card only. He switched to his card.

"I could have paid," Miriam said. It had been a trivial sum.

"I want half of it."

"How will eating half of my cookie work to relieve my stress?" She took a second package and waved her phone over the payment device. She handed the second cookie to him. They took an empty table and sat in silence. Eating and drinking.

"This isn't so bad," Sterling said, raising his coffee cup in a mock salute.

"That's because you are an uncultured American."

"Can you say that as a fellow American?"

"I said it on behalf of all Aussies," Miriam countered. "It's just how it is."

"I like instant coffee just fine. And so does Stephanie."

She slowly shook her head. "I can't even look at you right now."

"I wouldn't look at me, either. I'm an embarrassment. I lost Stephanie to a toad like Jeremy."

"And you won her back because you never stopped caring, although the stalking her on the cruise ship thing? That was a high-risk maneuver with the greatest probability of failure. Risk is my business, and I would have never advised that. But I, for one—and Stephanie, too—thank you for doing it."

"It's tearing me up inside," he admitted.

"Waiting is the hardest part," she agreed. They finished their cookies, finished their coffee, and picked up a second cup before heading out of the cafeteria. Jeremy was nowhere to be seen when they stepped into the corridor.

"I hope this means you've solved our Jeremy problem. I would be way okay to never see that dude again."

"You and me both. I fear that we haven't seen the last of him."

"Should we call the embassy?" Sterling asked out of the blue. He returned to the dining area, sat at the nearest table, and pulled out his phone.

Miriam thought for a moment. It wasn't her job to call them as an insurance representative, but she often did. "I have the number."

Sterling tapped it into his phone as she read it aloud. He slid her phone charging setup across the table to her.

The U.S. embassy operator picked up right away. "I'd like to report that a U.S. citizen is in emergency surgery. It's unknown if she'll pull through."

The operator took the details, apologizing that no one was there to speak with him directly.

He didn't have her passport number, but he had her name and social security number, which he gave them.

"I'll call when I know more," he promised.

"Why do you have her SSN?"

"I've done her taxes," Sterling replied. "I'm sure she wouldn't mind me telling the embassy since I don't have her passport. We never went anywhere requiring one." He stared into the distance. Regret. She had wanted to go somewhere exotic, but he didn't. He glanced at the faces of those taking a break from their work in the hospital. Determined and professional. Generally happy. He didn't know what it was like in the States. Were hospital employees there this gratified with their work and their working conditions?

The thoughts he had when he was trying not to think about Stephanie, but he couldn't focus. Not on one thing or another.

"Shall we?" Miriam pushed in her chair for a second time.

Sterling joined her and together, they headed for the stairs. Up one flight to the first floor and the waiting room, where they once again found themselves alone. No one was at the desk, either.

The wait that seemed like death by a thousand cuts. Sterling's heart hammered inside his chest. He had a hard time getting a full breath.

Miriam caught sight of him struggling. "It's a panic attack," she said. "You have to slow down, let the earth catch up with you, then plant your feet firmly on the ground."

He buried his face in his hands and focused on his breathing, which only made it harder.

Miriam rushed to the double doors and pounded on them. Soon enough, a nurse appeared. "Can I help you?"

"He's having a panic attack. I fear he's going to pass out," Miriam said.

"Wait here. I'll be right back." The nurse hurried away. She returned a minute later towing an oxygen tank hooked up with a regulator and mask. She kneeled next to Sterling. "Put this on."

She helped him adjust the mask. She turned the oxygen up about halfway, five liters per minute.

"Slow, deep breaths," she advised. Demonstrating breathing slowly while he panted until he slowed into a more normal rhythm. The nurse reduced the oxygen flow. After two minutes, he was breathing normally. She removed the mask. "How do you feel?"

"Better. Sorry for being so weak," he said softly.

"You're not weak. You care. If you didn't, then you wouldn't be panicking, now would you?" She smiled at him and prepared to return to the surgical area.

"Can you tell me, how is Stephanie doing?"

"Surgery is almost finished. I think they've done all they need to do. The doctor should be out shortly. Which reminds me, I better get a wheelchair for him." She rushed into the surgical area, dragging the wheeled tank with her.

"That's some good news," Miriam said. "Surgery is finished. We'll know more shortly, and that nurse knows to bring the surgeon out here. She would have never known to do that if you hadn't needed a couple minutes of her time."

"Thanks for beating down the door," he said, watching the window that showed the corridor leading into the surgical area. "She survived the surgery. That's a good sign."

"That's the best sign, Sterling." Miriam stood. She walked back and forth, not pacing but not wanting to sit down. She'd spent too much of her day in a chair already. That's what she liked about her job. She was on her feet for much of her workday when she visited hospitals.

But today was a different day, a hard day.

---

THE RESULTS WERE MIRACULOUS. Similar to squeezing pus from a nasty skin pimple, the relief of obstruction and drainage of pus had immediate effects on Stephanie's general condition. Her blood pressure increased, and her pulse decreased. Joe breathed a sigh of relief. Stephanie appeared to have come out of the woods. All this in just over twenty minutes of expert endoscopic surgery. Having the right surgeon made all the difference.

"What are we going to do with her gallbladder?" Bethany asked.

"I'll let her recover from the septic shock and cholangitis, and we can deal with the gallbladder in a day or two. We have averted the worst of it. I expect her to recover quickly."

# CHAPTER TWENTY-THREE – NEW LIFE

CHIP STRUGGLED TO GET into the wheelchair. The pain had grown almost intolerable, but he'd finished the two separate procedures—that was, if you included restarting the patient's heart after a crash.

Bethany was managing the clean-up of the operating room. Stephanie had been transferred straight to the intensive care unit to continue careful monitoring during her expected recovery. She remained in critical condition and was in a controlled coma. She would be reviewed later in the day and if her obs improved, she would be extubated.

Abby assisted Chip and Possum Joe took over as wheelchair driver.

"You should get that looked at," Joe insisted. He knew where he was taking Chip.

"Waiting room first," Chip said, lifting his head while attempting to relax his features from their pain-induced wince.

Joe diverted from his track toward the elevator to the corridor out of the surgical area and into the waiting room, where he found Miriam and Sterling.

"He's okay. You can tell us both," Miriam said.

It wasn't standard procedure, but Chip was too tired to argue. "She's stable but still in critical condition. We successfully removed the obstructing gallstone and drained the pus. She has been taken to the I.C.U. for recovery. We'll know in twelve to twenty-four hours how well she pulled through. She is under cardiac care, so they'll be ready if anything happens."

"Cardiac care?" Miriam wondered.

"What's wrong with her heart?" Sterling asked.

"She suffered cardiac arrest during the surgery, but through immediate defibrillation, normal heartbeat was restored. The toxins that entered her body have not yet cleared her system. That will take some time, but she's on the best medication to help her through it. I believe she'll fully recover, and that is my professional opinion." Chip was taking a risk, but he also had confidence that he had done his job well.

He also based his opinion on how quickly she returned from the crash. Her heart wasn't ready to stop beating yet. Sometimes, the reaper came for people too early. It was Chip's job to fight him off.

"Thank you," Sterling said and grasped Chip's hand, pumping it almost frantically. Sterling staggered back and flopped into a chair.

Miriam only smiled. "That's what we've been waiting what seems like a lifetime to hear. Thanks, Chip. If it's not too much to ask, why are you in a wheelchair?"

"Hit by a car running to get here. I'm off to the E.R. to see what the damage was. Push, Possum Joe, push." Chip waved his hand in the air and pointed toward the elevator down the corridor.

Miriam tipped her chin knowingly to Joe. A doctor's sacrifice for Stephanie's benefit. Someone would eventually tell her what Chip had done, but not today.

Joe pushed the wheelchair back into the surgical area to use the elevator that would deliver Chip into the E.R. and not at the admissions desk.

When they arrived, the staff was finishing up with the last wave of patients and just taking a break.

"What do we have here? Roll-a-doc?" the doctor on duty asked.

"Bill! Good to see you on duty. I think Chip needs a colonoscopy," Joe quipped.

"Not quite," Chip said, allowing himself to grimace once more. It hurt to sit. It hurt even more to stand. "Hit by a car on the way here. I might have a proximal femur fracture or maybe even a fracture of the femoral neck. If I'm really lucky, it'll be both."

"Have you checked in with admissions?" Bill asked. He waved down a nurse walking by. "Prep Number Three, and we'll need a hip x-ray on this pending patient."

She hurried away.

"You have to check in first. Do you think you're special?" Bill raised his eyebrows.

Chip showed his badge and then looked at it himself. "I wouldn't trust the guy in that picture, either. We'll be right back." Chip circled his hand in the air and pointed toward admissions, which was where he wanted to go in the first place, but Joe had a different idea. In the end, they went where Chip needed to be.

The admissions nurse scanned his badge, made a couple entries in the system, and sent them back into the E.R. She didn't bother escorting them since they knew the way.

"Thank you," Chip called over his shoulder. "Number Three, garçon."

"I think you're enjoying this just a bit too much," Joe said.

"I'll admit that I'm not enjoying this at all. I joke to make light of how much pain I'm in. Something is seriously wrong, and I think I may have exacerbated the injury."

Joe leaned close. "You saved a life today, Chip. You know you'd do it again. Just like I would, or Bethany, or Abby, or just about anyone else in this hospital."

"You're right. It's what I like about this job. We can fix people and then get fixed ourselves without having to leave. Bring me food! I've a curry at home with my name on it that I won't see until after I'm starved to death."

"Talking about home, have you called your wife?" Joe asked.

"I meant to, but we had to hurry."

"Uh-huh." Joe handed his phone to Chip.

"Nyla, it's me. I'm at the hospital. Surgery is done. My car is somewhere downtown, maybe. A couple kids stole my keys and my phone. I better call the police. Oh yeah, I was hit by a car and am in the emergency room getting an x-ray. I'll be home later."

The call ended after a robust diatribe that gave Chip no chance to say anything.

"I take it she's not happy?" Joe posited.

"A lot. Probably more than a lot. But she has the address where the phone is right now. You should be getting a text. There it is."

Chip studied the phone. He forwarded the address to his email. He gave the phone back to Joe. "A nice lady took a picture of the car that hit me and sent that to my email, too. I'll put together a package for the police as soon as I can get to my desk."

"What are you doing out here?" Bill asked. He gestured toward the examination room that had been designated for Chip. When he tried to stand to shift into the bed, he would have collapsed if it hadn't been for Joe and Bill catching him.

"Sorry, mate," Chip said, leaning heavily on the two younger men. They eased him into bed, adjusting it until Chip gave the thumbs-up. "That relieves most of the pain. It's just a dull throb now."

A nurse hooked Chip up to the blood pressure cuff and O2 sensor. She took his temperature. "Slightly elevated," she reported before noting it in the system.

"At least you didn't have that curry, otherwise you'd be boiling." Joe and Bill both laughed. Chip didn't see the humor because he was hungry, and that curry sounded like it would hit the spot. When Joe saw his face, he asked, "What?"

"I think Nyla is coming to the hospital."

"Should I tell her to bring your curry?" Joe laughed again.

A technician appeared with the portable x-ray machine.

"I don't mean right now. I mean coming to work here, in social services."

"Oh." Joe shrugged. "We better let the professionals do their job." Joe and Bill excused themselves while the technician placed the plate under Chip and lined up the machine to take a digital image. It was over in thirty seconds. The technician maneuvered the unit out of the room.

Joe and Bill reappeared.

"Since it's just a bruise or broken bone or something generally irrelevant, I've ordered you some food," Joe said.

Bill nodded. "He did."

"Do people get to eat in the E.R.? How long do you think I'm going to be here?"

"Once the x-ray confirms a fracture, probably a while. I don't think we'll be able to put you into a full-body cast, but maybe traction. What do you think, Joe?"

"Traction, definitely. Is the colonoscopy off the table?"

"Probably," Bill replied. "How old are you, Chip?"

"No colonoscopy. If I wanted one, I'd do it myself." Chip glanced from one doctor to the other, scolding them with just a look at their descent into other forms of humor and taking far too much pleasure in his discomfort. "It's not like I hurt myself sleeping or playing golf. I might deserve some ridicule in those cases. Not this one."

Joe winked at him. "You've been the ironman of the team, Chip. Let us have our fun. Do you want me to check in on Stephanie?"

"If you would. I'd go up there myself to make sure she's comfortable, but you know how it is. I have food coming." Chip winked back.

"I'll be back," Joe promised.

Bill excused himself to check on the x-ray and see what the radiologist had to say. No reading was final until a radiologist confirmed what it showed. Any other doctor could only make a preliminary reading, no matter how obvious the injury seemed.

Chip lay in the reclined bed, slightly raised with a pillow under his head. He could have used a drink of water. He wasn't worried. The call button was right there at the edge. He wanted to know how Stephanie was doing. He wanted to call his wife back. He needed to call the police. Too much to do to lounge in bed, even if it was in the emergency room. He tried to push himself upright, but that wasn't happening without a resurgence of the pain that put him there in the first place.

Relax, he counseled himself. It was hard to do because it seemed like he'd been running his whole life. One little injury wasn't going to stop him. He tried to prioritize everything he had to do, make it easier for when he was free, when Bill returned.

"Way to go," Bill started. "You do not have a fracture, but you have significant soft tissue damage. In the vernacular of yesterday's youth, you have one gnarly bruise. Why didn't you put ice on that? You wouldn't be in so much pain now if you'd taken care of it right away. Doctors! You make the worst patients." He watched for Chip to react, but he didn't. "Do you have any other surgeries you need to do today or tomorrow or maybe for the next month?"

"Not today. Tomorrow, yes, and almost every day thereafter," Chip replied. "I have a busy clinic."

"I figured. You're going to need pain pills and to minimize use of that leg. I recommend a cane when you have to walk, but try to minimize that. You take public transportation, don't you?"

Chip nodded.

"There's the double-edged sword, because what I'm prescribing you isn't anything you can take and then drive or operate. You take it at night to get some sleep, and then for maybe a couple more days. It's going to hurt, but it'll heal."

"Do you have any good news?"

"We know you weren't faking your pain, but you failed when it came to skeletal analysis. The shame! Congratulations! You're a doctor who's honest about his pain but incorrect about the cause."

Chip chuckled. That wasn't the answer he was looking for. He'd have to cut back on what he ate and not take in calories that he wasn't going to burn if he were to take it easy for a while.

"Your prescription is with the hospital pharmacy. You can pick it up there along with a cane, although if I were you, I'd get a sexy one from a store."

"There's such a thing as a sexy cane?" Chip asked.

"Have you never watched *The Avengers*? Someone of your age... Never mind."

"I'm not that old," Chip countered.

"We'll get you out of here after you've eaten." The doctor leaned out of the door and waved someone in. An orderly.

"DoorDash for Doctor Hips McClure?"

"That's Chip. My name is Chip."

"It definitely says Hips, but whatever. There you go, Doc." The lad handed it over and then disappeared into the corridor.

"Smells like curry." Bill sniffed the air demonstratively. "You have good friends, Hips."

"You are not calling me that. Possum Joe will be paid back for this, and the price will be high!" Chip looked around. "Where is he?"

# CHAPTER TWENTY-FOUR – APOGEE

JOE SHOWED HIS BADGE to the nurses at their station within the I.C.U., but none of them looked up as he walked by. He stopped when he realized intensive care was about half-full. Even with names on the outside of the doors, it would be easier to ask.

"Stephanie Trent?" He held his hands up and looked left and right.

"Twelve. That way." The nurse pointed. Her eyes never left her screen. Joe risked a glance. It was a medical record for one of the patients.

Chip had dictated while he operated, and the new AI-driven voice capture had recorded his version of the operation, including the immediate response to the crash. If Chip needed to add other notes, he could do that afterward, but for being incapacitated by his injury. The notes were already in the system. Efficiency that improved recordkeeping and saved the doctors' time.

Joe made a beeline for Room Twelve and found an orderly hovering over the still-unconscious patient. "Can I help you?" Joe asked.

"Moving the patient," the orderly replied.

"On whose orders? She needs to stay right here."

The orderly shrugged.

Joe returned to the nurses' station less than ten meters away. He tapped on the counter surrounding it. "Who ordered the patient in Number Twelve to be moved?"

"I don't know. I'll check."

She tapped a series of keys. "No one has. She's post-op on broad-spectrum antibiotics. Pulse and O2 are constant, and blood pressure is taken once every hour."

"Why is an orderly preparing to move her?"

"That's a good question." The nurse rose and walked straight for Room Twelve with Joe close on her heels.

The orderly had removed the cuff and oxygen sensor. He'd removed two of the ECG leads from Stephanie's chest.

"Leave those," the nurse ordered.

The orderly looked up.

"Where's your badge?" she asked.

He shrugged again. "Patient is being transferred," he said and returned to removing the leads. "Please bring the portable ventilator that is used for transfer of ventilated patients."

"Code Black," Joe nearly screamed. The nurse ran for her station to make sure the call was made to the entire hospital. "You need to stop."

"Can't do that, Doc. Stephanie and I are leaving. There's an ambulance waiting down below. She'll be well taken care of. You don't have to worry."

"I do worry because she's my friend's patient, and I'm not going to let her go without getting his order to move her." Joe grabbed the orderly's arm.

The orderly pulled away, and a scalpel appeared in his other hand. “You need to back off.”

Running feet pounded toward them.

“Leave her and go. No one will stop you,” Joe promised.

The security guard showed up. “Not you again. Jeremy. That’s your name, isn’t it?” he asked. “And with a weapon. I haven’t pounded a punk into next week in a good three or four days. I’m looking forward to this. Give us the room.” The guard nodded toward the door.

He pulled a small baton from his belt. It didn’t look like much of a weapon, but he inverted it and held it along his forearm. He raised his fists and eased forward.

Jeremy slashed an X in front of himself. He moved closer to Stephanie, keeping her between him and the guard. He pulled her IV away with his free hand. Then he followed a wire with his fingers to remove another lead from the ECG.

“We’re leaving and if you try to stop me, someone is going to get hurt, and it might not be either one of us.” He glanced toward Stephanie.

The security guard hesitated. “What do you want me to do?”

Joe looked around the area. A hospital was filled with potential weapons, but he’d never considered them as such. A rolling stand that a patient could use to drag an IV along with them while they walked. A metal tray for instruments or medications or meals.

The stand was heavy but not prohibitively so. Joe picked it up and wedged it under his armpit. He charged forward, grabbing a tray off the side table and tossing everything on it away. He dropped the tray across Stephanie’s mid-section and drove the stand forward, pushing Jeremy away from the patient.

The security guard moved around the bed now that Jeremy was clear of her, but Jeremy was fast. He ducked under the guard's reach and punched him hard, right on his belly button. The guard doubled over.

Joe rammed the stand's wheels into Jeremy's head, knocking him sideways.

The guard came up in a furor. He blocked Jeremy from Stephanie on his side of her bed, while Joe was on the other.

Jeremy looked for a way to her.

More feet pounded down the corridor.

Jeremy sidestepped, slashing at the nurse's face but not close to touching her. She stumbled backward and fell, screaming, and he bolted toward the second entrance to the I.C.U. The security guard lumbered after him.

Joe didn't wait. The patient needed him. He dropped the stand and removed the tray. He checked the ECG leads. The connectors were still attached to Stephanie's skin. They were color-coded, and all he had to do was clip the leads to the electrodes. He put the automatic BP cuff on her arm and lastly, clipped the O2 sensor on her finger. He checked her IV. It was firmly where it belonged. The drip was metered as Chip had directed.

There was no sign of the security guard, but two healthy young orderlies stood on either side of the nurse.

Her hand was shaking. "Secure the I.C.U. Make sure no one enters without a badge or your express authorization," Joe told her.

The I.C.U wasn't his domain. Doctors from all over the hospital had patients there for recovery or emergency treatment. They needed twenty-four-hour monitoring and regular delivery of medications.

In Stephanie's case, it was intravenous. Others received pills, if they were alert enough and could swallow freely. Others had nebulizer treatments for lung problems. Twenty-four-hour care of every type needed to help people to live.

Like Stephanie, who was the least deserving of everything that had befallen her. Joe rested his hand on her arm. "Little did we know that besides saving you from an attack inside your body, we had to deal with an attack outside, too. Westpark Hospital. We do it all."

Joe used the phone in the room to call the E.R. A nurse answered and transferred the call to Chip's room. She had to go to the room and answer it herself since he couldn't get up.

"It's Doctor Chambers," she said and handed Chip the phone.

"How's Stephanie?" Chip asked.

"She's doing just fine. Her numbers are looking better, but that guy, Jeremy is his name, was up here unhooking her. He said he had an ambulance to take her away. We chased him off after a little test of manliness. Did you get your food?"

"You're thinking about food after you have to fight off a man trying to steal our patient?"

"It's curry, Chip, and I can hear you eating. It's not just food, and there's no sense dwelling on the bad stuff in life, is there? We have additional security for Stephanie."

"Put out a PA call for Miriam Kiryakova and Sterling Bower. If we want security beside her bed, I bet Sterling will be more than happy to stay there all night."

"You know something I don't know, Hips?"

"You're going to pay for that, and why yes, I'm sure I know a lot of things you don't know. I bet you know tidbits I don't know either. How did you chase him away?"

"Jousting at the renaissance festival. I won my weight class."

"You did?" Chip was surprised. The nurse reappeared with two pills. Oxycodone. Enough to take the edge off his injured hip and leg.

"See? I did know something you didn't know. There are no weight classes, just two people trying to slam a big stick into each other's chest. It's exhilarating."

Chip downed the pills. "I'll take your word for it. Gotta go. My curry is getting cold."

"How are you getting home?" Joe asked before Chip could hand the phone back to the nurse.

"I haven't thought that far ahead."

"I'll give Nyla a call. Maybe we'll just put you in a taxi or an ambulance. How about an ambulance ride, Doctor?"

"My car is somewhere in the city," Chip countered.

"And you're in no shape to drive it, even if you did have your keys. I'm calling Nyla. Stay where you are and don't give the nurses any trouble." Joe hung up.

Less than a minute later, the public address asked Miriam and Sterling to report to the E.R. waiting room.

Chip finished his curry and set the empty package aside. He leaned back and closed his eyes. The next thing he knew, a rude voice was waking him.

"Good thing you ate. You're not supposed to take those pills on an empty stomach. Curry? Was that vindaloo? The whole of E.R. smells funny." Bill tsk-tsked.

Joe stood behind him with his arms crossed.

"Why don't you go home?" Chip said.

"Because I'm on shift," Bill replied.

"I think he meant me. I'm waiting for Nyla to get here. If she needs help with your sorry excuse for manhood, I'll go with her and make sure you get tucked in nice and tight."

Chip giggled. "With friends like you, who needs enemies?"

"Enemas? We're not giving those, but if we were, you'd be first in line." Joe's phone rang. He answered it but ended the call quickly. "Nyla is here. I'll bring her back."

When Joe returned, he had Nyla with him. "Sorry, honey," Chip started.

"I should be angry with you, but I'm not. I'm concerned, as any good spouse would be. How broken are you?"

"Just soft tissue damage, so I'll be good after a week? Maybe two days. Maybe a month," Chip joked.

"It'll take a while to heal, but he should be without pain in ten or eleven months," Bill offered.

"That long?" Nyla was shocked.

"He's kidding. They're poking fun at the broken old man." Chip shook his head.

Joe pulled Nyla aside. "He was a superhero today. Go easy on him, because the Lord knows, we aren't.

Everyone needs a friend like me who will give you a good kick when you're down, but not to keep you down, to bring you back up."

"Whatever that means. When are you going to find yourself a wife?"

Chip erupted with a hearty guffaw. "She gives as good as you get or something like that." He sobered. "Can I go home now?"

"Use your cane and don't be alone. I'll write you a note so you don't have to go to school tomorrow. You should probably take the whole week off. It's a bruise but a nasty one," Bill explained. "Doctors tend to make the worst patients. I'm going to put out a notice saying if anyone sees you in here, they're to report you to the director. I'm not kidding, Chip."

Chip leaned his head back and closed his eyes.

"He's not used to painkillers, is he?" Bill asked Nyla.

"No. He's used to toughing it out." She slowly shook her head while watching her husband. She checked his phone's location. "I'm calling the police while we let him take a little nap. I have the address where the phone is located. Maybe the police can recover his car keys, too."

Nyla made the call from within the room. Joe waited, too, even though he was under no obligation. It's what friends did for each other. If he had plans, they were canceled. He intended on giving Nyla and Chip a ride back to their house, which put him on the road for nearly three hours since he lived an hour in the other direction from the hospital. It was the least he could do, especially if Chip was going to have to reschedule his appointments for the week.

Bethany and Abby showed up. They were both in their street clothes while Chip and Joe were still in scrubs.

"There you are," Bethany said, but she quieted when she saw Nyla on the phone. She smiled, and they took each other's free hand for a moment. Joe took the nurses into the corridor to update them. As a doctor, his privacy was legally guaranteed. As a boss, he kept his team informed. He would have told them himself had he been awake.

"Can you stay here with them? I want to check with security to make sure they chased that Jeremy guy out of the building." The nurses shivered at the thought of someone trying to take a ventilated patient from the I.C.U.

Joe went to the waiting room first, where he found Miriam and Sterling pacing. New patients had arrived and were waiting to be seen. Another toddler coughing, and a man with a heavy bandage on his arm with blood soaking through.

In other words, the usual. It was Sunday, and do-it-yourself projects went awry with great frequency, and then there were the weekend illnesses to be addressed before Monday's return to school.

Joe stepped aside, where Miriam and Sterling joined him. "We found Jeremy in scrubs in the intensive care unit. He was attempting to remove Stephanie."

"What?" Sterling was shocked by the revelation. "Where is he?"

"I'm going to check on that now. Security was chasing him, last we saw. She's still in her room, and there is someone there with her, orderlies, but I was hoping you'd volunteer to stay with her."

"Consider it done," Sterling said without hesitation. "Where is she?"

"The I.C.U.," Joe replied, mildly confused since he'd already told him where she was.

"Of course. I'm going there now." He bolted for the stairs.

"Is there anything I can do?" Miriam wondered.

"She has nothing with her. She's not going back to the ship, and neither is Jeremy. Someone will have to collect her things, like a passport, ID, and what she'll need to leave the country, assuming she pulls through. She's still in bad shape."

"I'll call the embassy and work with Sterling to call the cruise line and anyone else who needs to step up. Plus, I hate to admit it, we're going to have a fight with the insurance company on what they'll cover. Did you know Sterling is a lawyer?"

"I don't know anything about any of you, except what Chip has told me."

Miriam smiled. "Sorry about that. You work for Chip?"

"*With* Chip. Doctor Joe Chambers, anesthesiology. These Neanderthals call me Possum Joe."

"Miriam Kiryakova, Unified International Healthcare. Nice to meet you." She handed him her card. "Stephanie. What a mess, huh?"

"I've seen less drama on daytime serials." He snorted his disbelief at the last two days but quickly sobered. "Keep your fingers crossed. We'll know more by tomorrow."

"I'll burn up the phone lines. I'll stay in touch with Chip and Sterling," she promised.

"Chip is out of it with his injury. You can call me. I'll text you so you have my number." He immediately pulled out his phone and typed the number on her card.

Miriam's phone buzzed. The text was simple. *Call me Joe.*

She saved his number under Doctor Joe and waved. She walked away slowly, looking back to see if he watched her leave, which he did. Once she was gone, he returned to the E.R. to find Bethany and Abby helping Nyla get Chip ready to go.

"That's it, huh? You're abandoning us?" Joe winked at Nyla before picking up the phone and checking in with the I.C.U.

"That man outside... His name is Sterling, and I sent him to sit with Stephanie. He'll be good for her. On my authority, Doctor Chambers, let him stay with her. It's the best therapy we can think of to get her through the hardest part of this. How is she?"

Joe nodded as he listened.

"Thank you," he said before hanging up. "Chip, she's stable. Blood pressure is normal."

"Some good news, then." Chip finished dressing. He leaned heavily on his hospital-provided cane.

"I'll drive," Joe told them.

"You don't have to. We'll grab an Uber, a van-sized one so Chip has room to stretch out," Nyla replied. "You have a sports car, don't you?"

"Well, yes, but there's a back seat." Joe hadn't thought it all the way through.

"I appreciate your big heart, but you go home, too. All of you," Nyla looked pointedly at Chip's team. "Your patient is in good hands. Trust the I.C.U."

"Hear, hear," Joe said. "If you need anything, don't hesitate to call. I mean anything, like someone to eat Chip's curry since he can't have anything solid for at least four days."

"They didn't say anything like that with the discharge instructions," Nyla countered.

"Don't listen to him," Chip interjected. "He tried to get me a colonoscopy when I reported to the E.R."

# CHAPTER TWENTY-FIVE – INSURANCE

MIRIAM LOOKED AT HER screen. The initial response was a complete rejection of all claims due. She had submitted a preliminary request to gauge the response, and now she had it.

She hung her head. This was in no way final, but it portended a fight. She dialed her phone.

"Sterling here. Be quick. Phone's about to die."

"Initial claim rejected. Fight's on."

"That's downright inconvenient," Sterling replied in a tired voice. "Stephanie is doing better. Fever's down. She has been extubated and mumbled something unintelligible. I'm not sure she was awake." The phone went dead.

"Get a new phone with some battery life!" Miriam shouted, even though Sterling was already gone. She'd have to go to the hospital to find out more about Stephanie. Sterling sounded as upbeat as possible, considering he had been up all night. The stress of it all had to be exhausting.

Miriam had slept well. She'd have to check in with Chip to get the inside information on Possum

Joe. He was a little bit older. Maybe that was a good thing. The younger men she dated tended to have insecurities that they projected onto anyone they liked. Doctor John had potential, too, but neither man was going to be graced with her presence until she resolved the billing concerns of her client.

It was an injustice that she wasn't going to allow. She checked the time. It was seventeen hours earlier. She was used to adding seven hours to her current time but knowing that it meant yesterday. It was mid-afternoon at their headquarters in the States.

She called the man who moved her into her position, the one-and-only Herford Hartz. He was a legend in the industry, gifted for bridging the gap between corporate concerns and clients. The insured wanted everything paid for, while the shareholders wanted no outflow but also happy clients willing to continue contributing to the bottom line.

That meant more people without problems buying policies. That's where Herford excelled. Marketing insurance protection to people who had a minimal chance of needing it. Harp on the exceptions. Make them sound the norm. And then tout a discount. Get more for less. The clientele had grown by millions.

This made Unified International a very big company with massive dividends for shareholders.

That's why stock options were so attractive. Shareholder value. It took a good salary and made it great.

She was on the cusp.

But Stephanie. Fighting the company wasn't a winning strategy. She needed advice. She called his direct number. He picked up on the fourth ring.

"How's my favorite liaison doing in the delightful summer in the land down under?" He had a way of making everyone feel special.

"It's getting nice down here. I have a question about dealing with a rejected claim." She let the non-question hang in the air.

"You let the client down gently with the facts of their policy. They'll claim they were misled, and you show them their contract with initials on each provision, specifically the one that was rejected. You're the liaison, though. You have locals to handle that for you. That's the beauty of our international coverage."

Miriam looked at her phone. Her mentor had missed her point in entirety. "I've taken a personal interest in this case. A passenger on a cruise ship. Gallstones that sent her to the E.R. but weren't bad enough for surgery so she went back to sea and then they got really bad. Medevaced to the hospital via helicopter and surgery later. I believe she's on the mend, but she almost died."

"Hmm. Sounds like you've gotten too close to the client."

"Stephanie. Her name is Stephanie," Miriam interrupted.

"And she's our client. I'm sure there are nuances that apply in her case. Find them, make an offer, and move on."

"I have a lawyer looking into it, Stephanie's boyfriend."

There was a long silence, so long that Miriam checked her phone to see if they were still connected.

"You brought in outside counsel?"

"He's her boyfriend. She shouldn't be bankrupted because of the coverage gap between a policy upgrade."

"After she felt better, she upgraded her policy, even though that was now a pre-existing condition?"

"I did it for her," Miriam admitted. She felt like she was in elementary school telling the principal that she pulled angry Betty's hair.

"You probably shouldn't have done that. You put the company on the hook when there's no way we would have approved an upgrade, which is why the gap exists, to catch errors like this. Does she know about any of this?"

"No. She's still in the I.C.U, from what I understand." Miriam was as uncomfortable as she'd ever been. Herford's tone had changed. He sounded cold and was growing more distant. "But her boyfriend..."

"Yes. The boyfriend. What kind of costs are we looking at?"

"I guess it'll be upwards of a quarter of a mil Australian, which is about one-eighty U.S."

"That's a big number." Herford whistled between his teeth. "I feel responsible in that I set you up for this and set you up to fail. I can personally approve this, but you'll be finished. If you defend the company and let her know she has limited coverage and then want to reduce costs, negotiate with the hospital as you've been doing, then we can make believe this never happened, and you can learn a valuable lesson."

"That's a hard choice," Miriam admitted.

"It's not, really. Loyalty to the company goes a long way." Herford was unflinchingly candid. "And loyalty to me."

"I understand. Take care of business, and I'll take care of you."

The job had always been one of taking care of the clients in a way that worked for both the company and the client, who always wanted one hundred percent of the bill covered, which almost never happened. When costs for the company rose, the client suffered.

Was she ready to accept that? From the inside, she could protect the next person and the one after that. If she was let go, she couldn't help anyone. If she was let go, she'd have to leave Australia immediately, because her business visa would be revoked, ending her status to legally stay in the country.

"I'll have to call you back," she said.

"If you hang up, then I'll know you've made your choice. I'll cover your client for you, but you can start packing your bags."

"Hardball. Is that what we are now? I've learned a great deal from this. And in just a few minutes, I've learned that the man I thought I knew as my mentor saw me as a tool. I helped the company's bottom line, but the second we deviate from that, it's the end of days! The sky is falling, and the world is ending. This one payout won't affect shareholder value one iota. A public lawsuit showing how the company put the client last would destroy the marketing campaign which touts the client first and foremost. That's why you're willing to write this one off. Your answer is, do it, for me, please. And by the time you've clicked the box, you'll have my resignation."

Miriam was shaking. It took her three tries to click 'end' on the call.

From stock options to the unemployment line at the speed of a single phone call. The first thing she did was check her bank account. She'd been socking money away, so she had enough to survive for a while, but she couldn't afford to pay for this apartment for very long without digging deep into her savings. She was supposed to leave the country soon, though. How long did she have once her visa was canceled?

Was it worth it? She didn't even know Stephanie.

She called Sterling before remembering that his phone had died. She called the I.C.U. and asked to be connected with Room Twelve.

Sterling answered.

"How is she?"

"Getting better with each minute. The doctor just stopped by on his rounds, and he was extremely positive. I think we've made it, thank God."

"Thank all the good people that worked to get us here, and Stephanie for fighting. She wants a life she can enjoy, and if I'm any judge of women, she wants to enjoy it with you. You two make a good couple."

"You're very kind, but Jeremy is out there somewhere. I may have to take up karate."

"I understand your concern. You'll have to watch your backs. I'll report him to the embassy, especially that little stunt with threatening a doctor and attempting to kidnap Stephanie right out of the I.C.U. He's completely lost his mind."

"I didn't work on the legal brief at all. I couldn't concentrate and no charger for my phone, but mostly worried about Steph."

"It's okay. I think you still need to prepare the brief, but I've gotten the charges covered."

"You did? You're a wizard. What did that take?"

"It cost me my job. Do you know anyone who is hiring?"

"Oh, man, Miriam. I'm so sorry."

"Don't be. It was a noble cause. I went out on top, defending a maiden's honor from any who would cause her grief."

Sterling smacked his lips. "What did you do to Jeremy?"

"Football. I told you already."

"I don't know what that means," he replied.

"Foot. Ball...or maybe balls."

"Oh. That would send a man like him into Never-never-land. Good on you. I might have to hire you as private security, just until I learn enough karate."

"Funny. I have to go. I better polish up my resume before they cut off all my access. As a matter of fact, this is a company phone. It'll probably get shut off pretty soon. I better call and get the billing changed over to my name. I'm also supposed to leave Australia. My visa will be canceled."

"We can all fly out together. Me, you, and Steph. Escape this madness by going home."

"Don't have one of those, but I'll do something. I'll stop by the hospital later. I have a lot of little things to do."

Miriam put her phone down and stared out the window of her condo. She was in no shape to move. She'd collected more clothes than was reasonable.

She had touched up some of the decorations, and much of what was inside was hers. Pack the clothes into boxes since only a small portion of it would fit into her luggage. Pack her luggage with multi-use outfits.

She was good at her job—client liaison and the intricacies of the insurance system—but if she looked for a new job with an insurance company, she'd find much of the same.

She threw some clothes in her suitcases but stopped before she gained any packing momentum.

Miriam called Joe. He answered on the first ring. "Hey! The hot chick called me first."

"*The hot chick*. Very nice. No wonder you're a bachelor."

"Ouch, that cuts me deep. Before you ask, I haven't heard from Chip."

"Actually, my question was a little more selfish," she started.

"Why yes, I am free for dinner, although I was talking with John from the E.R. and he thinks he might be doing dinner with you, so we're going to cross swords at high noon and fight for the honor of your hand."

"Are all men little boys?"

"At heart, yes. I interrupted. You have a question?"

"Is the hospital looking for an outreach coordinator or liaison of some sort?"

"Why would you ask that? What happened, Miriam?" Joe's voice turned from carefree to concerned in an instant.

"I no longer work for Unified International, and I'm not quite ready to leave Australia. I need a job."

"You'll have to tell me the story over dinner. In between, I'll ask the hospital's chief exec what's available. I'll get back with you. First, do you have Nyla's number?"

"I just have Chip's," she replied, but his phone had been stolen. "I better get Nyla's to check in on my favorite surgeon."

"I'll text it to you." He ended the call. The text came through with Nyla's number, along with a time and a restaurant name that she was unfamiliar with. Sydney was a big city. She looked it up. The other side of town and no expense account to charge it to.

She sighed. *I guess this is how the other half lives.* She looked up light rail and bus routes. Once she had one she could live with, she returned to packing, which was the last thing she wanted to do. Tears streamed down her face until she put on a playlist of breakup music, wrapped around the core of an old Taylor Swift album.

# CHAPTER TWENTY-SIX – LIFE MOVES ON

NYLA ENDED THE MOST recent call. She was a social butterfly and received numerous calls during the day, but nothing like today. Anyone and everyone had been in touch to give their best wishes.

Chip lounged in his recliner, which he newly considered the best purchase he'd ever made. It was the only place he had any relief from pain without being medicated.

"Who was that?" he asked.

"That was your insurance agent, Miriam Kir-something. She wanted to wish you the best, while also asking if you needed a social media manager or community liaison or secretary or anything would do."

"Why did she ask that?"

"She needs a job," Nyla replied.

Chip thought about that. She had a job, didn't she? Maybe not anymore. It was a long weekend for her. He could see where she might have overstepped her boundaries by caring about a patient. She was the kind of person everyone needed in their life.

"Call the CEO," Chip said.

"Please," Nyla reminded him. She couldn't wait until the police returned Chip's phone. They'd recovered it and his car keys from a fourteen-year-old's house. His father saw to it that everything was returned with promises of other reparations if needed. Nyla declined to press charges, assuming the boy had learned his lesson. Maybe he wouldn't, but someone else would have to push that issue.

The hit-and-run, though. That was something completely different. Chip had pulled up the email with the pictures of the vehicle and the license plate. Nyla forwarded those to the police, too, but she hadn't heard anything back.

Nyla pressed the speed dial number for the hospital. They transferred her to the CEO's secretary. She gave him that phone.

"Trevor, please. This is Chip McClure."

"One moment," the pleasant voice replied.

"Chip! You gave us quite the scare. I don't like seeing my doctors in wheelchairs."

"Were you there yesterday? I'm sorry I missed you."

"Actually, no. I don't like hearing from people who see my doctors in wheelchairs."

"Me neither, Trevor. I have a question. Miriam Kiryakova needs a job, and she is incredible liaising with patients. We have to have something for her. I'm pulling in a favor, if that's okay."

"You don't have to pull in a favor on that. I've already asked the board to look into it. We've been considering an outreach manager for the hospital's image. Although we'd prefer an Australian, there is a certain international skillset that is hard to find locally, even in a city with such diverse talent as

Sydney. And you're the second person to ask about her. Joe Chambers called earlier."

"Don't let me waste any more of your time. I was impressed with her work ethic and sheer determination."

"People have nothing but good to say about her. That's strange for an insurance agent. There's always that one person who's dissatisfied with everything and is the most vocal about it. The squeaky wheel and all that."

"Thanks, Trev. I'll go back to recuperating. Another couple days and I should be fine to come back to work."

"I'm no doctor—well, I am, but not that kind of doctor—but I'm pretty sure you won't be fine in two days. Pass my congratulations to Nyla on her new role as a counselor with our social work initiative."

Chip had the phone on speaker because he didn't like holding it to his head. He glanced over the top of it at his wife. She shrugged and disappeared into the kitchen.

"You're the best, Trev. I'll see you soon enough."

"Let me know when you're back and I'll stop down."

"I promise," Chip said.

"Which means you'll forget. I'll ask Bethany to call me."

"She won't forget." Both men knew that beyond a shadow of a doubt. Chip hung up. "When were you going to tell me?" he called.

"When I take you to work and stay there," she replied, her voice edgy because of shouting from the kitchen.

"I'd come out there and give you a big hug and a kiss, but I'm old and broken."

---

JOE HEADED UPSTAIRS. HE decided to walk because he had time to kill. With all Chip's surgeries delayed, Joe found himself without any patients to put under. He'd told other surgeons he was available, but every surgery already had an anesthetist assigned.

Bored. He liked being busy at work. This was his second visit to the I.C.U. over the course of four hours. The first time, he'd brought a phone charger for Sterling. This time, he was bringing a sandwich. Sterling hadn't asked for anything, but Miriam had asked a favor, and it was an easy one to grant.

In Stephanie's room, he found Sterling sitting and holding her hand, which he'd been doing for twenty-four hours straight.

"You holding up okay?" Joe asked.

"They brought me a recliner. I can try to get some sleep."

"I hate to be the bearer of bad news, but you look awful."

"I feel pretty good, though. Stephanie's getting stronger by the minute. Hey!" he nearly shouted when she squeezed his hand. "There you are." He leaned close while her eyelids fluttered until her eyes opened. "Gave us quite a scare, pretty lady."

"Hospital?"

"Westpark. They brought you back to life."

"I'm so happy to wake up and see you instead of Jeremy."

"Shh. Don't say his name. Don't give him any more power over you," Sterling said. "Whatever you need, I'm here for you."

Joe waited while the two looked at each other, and their conversation paused.

"Hi, Stephanie. We've met, but you weren't conscious. I'm Joe. I'm on Chip's surgical team, and I don't think I could be happier to see you open your eyes."

"Chip. I remember him."

"He's got that kind of face," Joe said. "Keep getting stronger. I hear there's a plane ticket with your name on it to take you home, but you'll need to stay here for a bit longer so we can monitor your heart."

"What's with my heart? It was my gallbladder," Stephanie wondered, confusion filling her face.

"Your heart stopped, but we gave it a nudge with a little electrical stimulation, and it started beating again. You were only down for three minutes. Welcome back to your new life."

"Wow. I died?"

"Not on our watch. You lived, and you're on the mend. Chip put in your record that we need to observe you for a while longer until we're sure you're healthy enough to travel, and then you go home. You still have your gallbladder, which is going to cause you more problems. We'll forward your record to your doctor so you can get that taken care of back home, first thing. You're young and strong. You'll get through all of this and be better for it."

"I don't know what to say, but you're right. I'm tired. Staying here for a while longer will be okay." Stephanie closed her eyes.

"I'll leave you to it." Joe excused himself. The first thing he did in the corridor was call Nyla and ask her to put Chip on.

"Chip. Your patient's awake. I thought you'd like to know."

***The end of A Surgeon's Dilemma***

Please leave a review on this book as well as the whole series, because all those stars look great and help others decide if they'll enjoy this book as much as you have. I appreciate the feedback and support. Reviews buoy my spirits and stoke the fires of creativity.

**Books in my Medical Thriller series**

A Surgeon's Dilemma – **https://geni.us/MedicalThriller**

A Surgeon's Peril – **https://geni.us/MedicalThriller2**

Don't stop now! Keep turning the pages as I talk about this book, as well as life in the sub-arctic.

You can always join my newsletter at https://craigmartelle.com or follow me on Amazon so you can be notified when my next book is published.

# Author Notes - Craig Martelle

*Written December 26th, 2025*

Thank you for reading! We hope you liked it. The fact that you're reading this means you are one in a billion! That's how many readers of English there are in the world. And you've chosen this book to invest the most precious of commodities—your time. This book came about for something to do while I was avoiding yet another Fairbanks winter.

My lungs are damaged from twenty years of mistreatment of asthma while serving in the U.S. Marine Corps. It's gotten so bad that the extreme cold is life threatening, that my lungs will seize up and I'll stop breathing altogether. I'm going to avoid that from now to forever. Good thing I chose this year to start saving myself. This December has been brutally cold with ambient temperatures clawing their way downward to -53F/-47C. Violently cold.

That's the foundation on why I'm not in Alaska while my wife and good boy Stanley stayed behind to manage the house and my wife is a professor at the university and kind of has to be there.

What to do while in Australia for three months? Writing a book was a given, but what was unique that could bring local talent into play, especially, my son's father-in-law who is a world-renowned surgeon. I asked Jim if he'd like to co-write a book with me based on a concept I floated, and he was all in!

I figured it would take two months with a certain amount of back and forth, but it only took 25 days to write this whole story. Jim was great with ideas and technical information. We worked a flowing, intertwining plot that I think worked. If you're still reading, then it definitely worked.

There were interesting points of contention, not from me, mind you, but one in particular. I called the public transport system in Sydney trams because that's what they're called in Adelaide, but that was completely wrong. They're the light rail, which was easily corrected. I didn't know, but then we got down to what are the individual vehicles called. Trains, trams, or light rail. People from Sydney gave us all three answers.

If you're from Sydney and you're reading this, be not so quick to condemn the use of the word tram because there are some of your fellows who call the cars that, while others call them trains, and still others refer to the vehicles by the bigger name of light rail. I'm probably the least caring out of all who engaged in this conversation. I just want to get it right. Turns out, there is no right answer. I guess it depends on a bunch of other factors, none of which I'm privy to.

Just tell me which word to use!

Sorry, can't do that.

Tram it is, those vehicles used on the light rail. Because they are technically trams. In Russian, they are called tramvay, which is for a vehicle that runs on rails inside a city but above ground connected to an overhead power supply. So the question of whether light rail has trains or trams will remain forever unanswered except by those with an opinion on the matter regarding what buffoons we are to stake our claim on such an important issue.

Calling it a car was right out. The light rail vehicle sounded misanthropic, a veritable attack on humanity itself. In any case, that was one of only a few variations on the conversation. If you have an opinion on the matter, don't hesitate to share it where I will compile them to show how many different opinions there are without a single and definitive answer.

We'll claim colloquial use for the unanswerable and be done with it.

But it gave us something to do and we're both proud of how the story turned out. Thank you again for reading. Stay tuned for more regarding the next book in this which was supposed to be a standalone but because of the wild success of this first book, we're working on another which may already be done, depending on when you've come on board with these medical thrillers.

**Characters**

Surgeon – Doctor Chip McClure and his wife Nyla, son Phillip and daughter Eugenia

Anesthetist/Anesthesiologist – "Possum" Joe Chambers

Operating Room Nurse – Bethany Smart, RN

Anesthetic Nurse – Abby Rennie

Stephanie Trent – patient, blocked bile duct

Jeremy Dissick – Stephanie's current boyfriend

Sterling Bower – Stephanie's ex-boyfriend

Miriam Kiryakova – Unified International Healthcare Insurance (614723)

Doctor Van Liet from the ship

Thank you for joining us for this story.

Peace, fellow humans.

---

**If you liked this story, you might like some of my other books.** You can join my mailing list by dropping by my website, or if you have any comments, shoot me a note at craig@craigmartelle.com. I am always happy to hear from people who've read my work. I try to answer every email I receive.

Also, please write a short review for me on Amazon. I greatly appreciate any kind words; even one or two sentences go a long way. The number of reviews an ebook receives greatly improves how well it does on Amazon.

Amazon—https://www.amazon.com/author/craigmartelle

Facebook—https://www.facebook.com/authorcraigmartelle

BookBub—https://www.bookbub.com/authors/craig-martelle

My web page—https://craigmartelle.com

Thank you for joining me on this incredible journey.

**Other Series by Craig Martelle**

**#—available in audio, too**

(#) (co-written with Michael Anderle)—a post-apocalyptic paranormal adventure

**Gateway to the Universe** (#) (co-written with Justin Sloan & Michael Anderle)—this book transitions the characters from the Terry Henry Walton Chronicles to the Bad Company

**The Bad Company** (#) (co-written with Michael Anderle)—a military science fiction space opera

**Judge, Jury, & Executioner** (#)—a space opera adventure legal thriller

**Shadow Vanguard**—a Tom Dublin space adventure series

**Superdreadnought** (#)—an AI military space opera

**Metal Legion** (#)—a military space opera

**The Free Trader** (#)—a young adult science fiction action-adventure

**Cygnus Space Opera** (#)—a young adult space opera (set in the Free Trader universe)

**Darklanding** (#) (co-written with Scott Moon)—a space Western

**Mystically Engineered** (co-written with Valerie Emerson)—mystics, dragons, & spaceships

**Metamorphosis Alpha**—stories from the world's first science fiction RPG

**The Expanding Universe**—science fiction anthologies

**Zenophobia** (#) (co-written with Brad Torgersen)—a space archaeological adventure

**Battleship Leviathan** (#)– a military sci-fi spectacle published by Aethon Books

**Glory** (co-written with Ira Heinichen)—hard-hitting military sci-fi

**Black Heart of the Dragon God** (co-written with Jean Rabe)—a sword & sorcery novel

**Starship Lost** – a hard-science, military sci-fi epic published by Aethon Books

**Veracity of Failure** – a hard-science technothriller, the race to Mars

**I, Soldier** – military sci-fi

**End Times Alaska** (#)—a post-apocalyptic survivalist adventure published by Permuted Press

**Nightwalker** (a Frank Roderus series)—A post-apocalyptic Western adventure

**End Days** (#) (co-written with E.E. Isherwood)—a post-apocalyptic adventure

**Successful Indie Author** (#)—a nonfiction series to help self-published authors

**Monster Case Files** (co-written with Kathryn Hearst)—A Warner twins mystery adventure

**Rick Banik** (#)—Spy & terrorism action-adventure

**Ian Bragg Thrillers** (#)—a hitman with a conscience

<u>Published exclusively by Craig Martelle, Inc</u>

**The Gygax Odyssey** – Luke Gygax and J. Clifton Slater – son of the legendary co-creator of Dungeons & Dragons™ retells the stories his father used to tell about the origin of the Gygax family

**A Couples Travels**—a nonfiction travel series

**Love-Haight Case Files** by Jean Rabe & Donald J. Bingle—the dead/undead have rights, too, a supernatural legal thriller

**Mischief Maker** by Bruce Nesmith—the creator of Elder Scrolls V: Skyrim brings you Loki in the modern day, staying true to Norse mythology (not a superhero version)

For a complete list of Craig's books, stop by his website—https://craigmartelle.com

Made in the USA
Monee, IL
13 September 2026

62976620R00154